Dear MyCopy Customer,

This Springer book is a monochrome print version of the eBook to which your library gives you access via SpringerLink. It is available to you at a subsidized price since your library subscribes to at least one Springer eBook subject collection.

Please note that MyCopy books are only offered to library patrons with access to at least one Springer eBook subject collection. MyCopy books are strictly for individual use only.

You may cite this book by referencing the bibliographic data and/or the DOI (Digital Object Identifier) found in the front matter. This book is an exact but monochrome copy of the print version of the eBook on SpringerLink.

Lecture Notes in Medical Informatics

Vol. 1: Medical Informatics Europe 78. Proceedings 1978. Edited by J. Anderson. XI, 822 pages. 1978.

Vol. 2: D. Fenna, S. Abrahamsson, S. O. Lööw and H. Peterson, The Stockholm County Medical Information System. VI, 163 pages. 1978.

Vol. 3: Long-Term Studies on Side-Effects of Contraception – State and Planning. Symposium 1977. Edited by U. Kellhammer and K. Überla. VI, 240 pages. 1978.

Vol. 4: Clinical Trials in 'Early' Breast Cancer. Proceedings 1978. Edited by H. R. Scheurlen, G. Weckesser and I. Armbruster. VI, 283 pages. 1979.

Vol. 5: Medical Informatics Berlin 1979. Proceedings 1979. Edited by B. Barber, F. Grémy, K. Überla and G. Wagner. XXIII, 970 pages. 1979.

Vol. 6: Health Care Technology Evaluation. Proceedings, 1978. Edited by J. Goldman. VII, 118 pages. 1979.

Vol. 7: Technology and Health: Man and his World. Proceedings, 1978. Edited by G. Wagner, P. L. Reichertz and E. Masè. VI, 243 pages. 1980.

Vol. 8: Mathematical Aspects of Computerized Tomography. Proceedings 1980. Edited by F. Natterer. VIII, 309 pages. 1981.

Vol. 9: Computers and Mathematical Models in Medicine. Proceedings, 1977. Edited by D. Cardús and C. Vallbona. VIII, 315 pages. 1981.

Vol. 10: B. Fries, Applications of Operations Research to Health Care Delivery Systems. V, 107 pages. 1981.

Vol. 11: Medical Informatics Europe 81. Proceedings 1981. Edited by F. Grémy, P. Degoulet, B. Barber, and R. Salamon. XXIII, 975 pages. 1981.

Vol. 12: G. Wiederhold, Databases for Health Care. VI, 75 pages. 1981.

Vol. 13: The Computer and Blood Banking. Proceedings, 1981. Edited by J. R. Möhr and A. Kluge. X, 275 pages. 1981.

Vol. 14.: F. Wingert, Medical Informatics. X, 247 pages. 1981.

Vol. 15: Digital Image Processing in Medicine. Proceedings 1981. Edited by K. H. Höhne. VIII, 197 pages. 1981.

Vol. 16: Medical Informatics Europe 82. Proceedings, 1982. Edited by R.R. O'Moore, B. Barber, P.L. Reichertz, and F. Roger. XX, 938 pages. 1982.

Vol. 17: Biomedical Images and Computers. Proceedings, 1980. Edited by J. Sklansky and J.-C. Bisconte. VII, 332 pages. 1982.

Vol. 18: D.P. Pretschner, Engymetry and Personal Computing in Nuclear Medicine. V, 129 pages. 1982.

Lecture Notes in Medical Informatics

Edited by D. A. B. Lindberg and P. L. Reichertz

18

D. P. Pretschner

Engymetry and Personal Computing in Nuclear Medicine

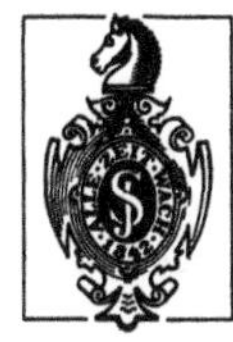

Springer-Verlag
Berlin Heidelberg GmbH 1982

Editorial Board

J. Anderson J. H. van Bemmel M. F. Collen S. Kaihara A. Levy
D.A.B. Lindberg (Managing Editor) H. Peterson A. Pratt
P. L. Reichertz (Managing Editor) W. Spencer C. Vallbona

Author

D.P. Pretschner
Department Radiologie,
Abteilung IV: Nuklearmedizin und spezielle Biophysik
Medizinische Hochschule Hannover
Karl-Wiechert-Allee 9, D-3000 Hannover 61, FRG

DOI 10.1007/978-3-642-93220-5

This work is subject to copyright. All rights are reserved, whether the whole or part of the material is concerned, specifically those of translation, reprinting, re-use of illustrations, broadcasting, reproduction by photocopying machine or similar means, and storage in data banks. Under § 54 of the German Copyright Law where copies are made for other than private use, a fee is payable to "Verwertungsgesellschaft Wort", Munich.

© by Springer-Verlag Berlin Heidelberg 1982
Originally published by Springer-Verlag Berlin Heidelberg New York in 1982
MyCopy version of the original edition 1982

2145/3140-543210
www.springer.com/mycopy

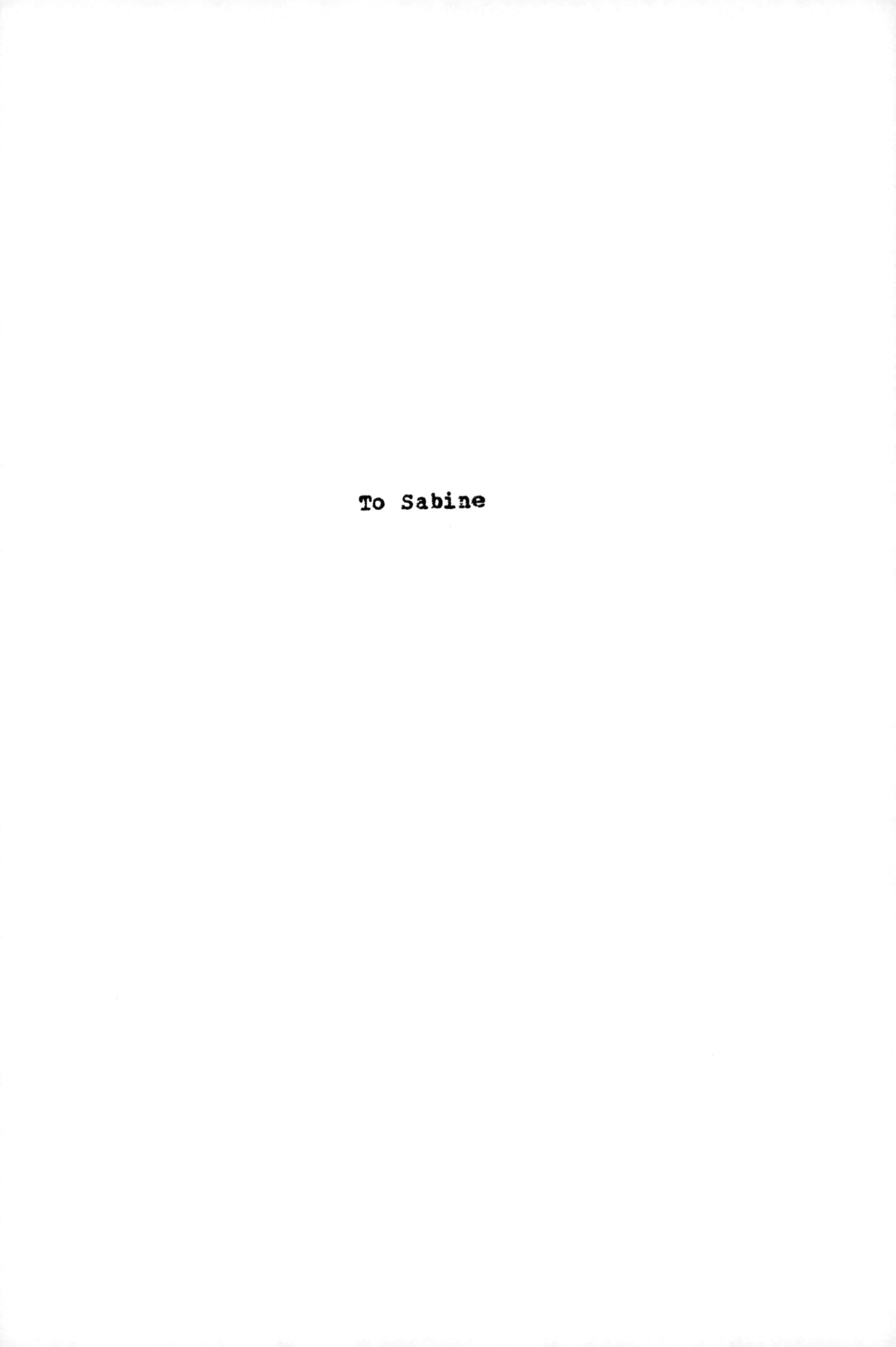

To Sabine

FOREWORD

Nuclear Medicine is not and has not been a purely imaging discipline. It is function analysis that has always been the focal point. This fact has become particularly obvious in the last few years through the employment of new short-lived radionuclides, new technical procedures and data processing. The disadvantage of function analysis in Nuclear Medicine through the use of radioactively labeled compounds is that more and more complicated and expensive equipment has to be used. A further characteristic is that these machines are stationary, and that the patients cannot be examined under physiological conditions. For technical reasons the γ-camera is developing in the direction of measuring mainly the so-called 'soft' γ-emitters at the present time. On the other hand, positron emitters are the radionuclides which are of interest for metabolic functions. At present, positron cameras are even more expensive and complicated machines, the use of which is very demanding.

In this book Priv.-Doz. Dr. med. Dipl.-Ing. D. Peter Pretschner has described a new system which contains his ideas and his technical developments. He describes a solution to the urgent questions and difficulties in the employment of radioactive substances for diagnosis. It does not demand large resources and can be used under the appropriate individual physiological conditions. Here he was helped by his training as a natural scientist and engineer, as well as by his being an experienced clinician. In my opinion, the procedure for diagnosis through Nuclear Medicine put forward by Dr. Pretschner opens up a new dimension, in particular with regard to the focal point of Nuclear Medicine: function analysis. His idea of localising the smallest possible radiation detectors at the decisive points on and in the patient, of storing the data in an appropriate memory, and of evaluating this data elsewhere after the examination period has, in fact, been realised by him after long and numerous tests. The decisive step for the success of this system, however, was the creation of relevant software within a personal computer system that had to be as compact as possible. For this purpose Dr. Pretschner has developed a new dialog language, with which it is possible to interpret mathematically complex analyses of measurement curves in a simple manner.

The results described in this book combine the technical know-how, which has been applied to and has solved the medical problems, with complicated methods of informatics. These results have produced a medical examination technique which opens up new aspects and possibilities for the future. The author must be congratulated on this achievement, and thanked on behalf of the patients and practical medicine.

Heinz Hundeshagen

ACKNOWLEDGMENTS

My grateful thanks are due to Professor Dr. P.L. Reichertz for his constant, encouraging support. He made it possible for me to take advantage of the comprehensive facilities of his outstanding department of Medical Informatics. I am grateful for many discussions with members of his staff, especially for the valuable comments of V. Spormann.

I wish to express my gratitude to Professor Dr. H. Hundeshagen for his continuing interest and support. The stimulating environment of his department of Nuclear Medicine and Special Biophysics promoted the development of MIESSY.

I have been extremely fortunate in receiving so much assistance from U. Gettner. The primary storage devices could not have reached the present stage of development without his excellent and constructive work. In addition I am indebted to H. Klee who assisted greatly in programming the personal computer system.

The clinical work of my colleagues Professor Dr. Th. Wuppermann, Drs. W.F. Schoener, V. Echtermeyer and of E.R. Kuse, D. R. Kiessling, W. Brenneisen contributed significantly to this book.

The technical help of G. Mueller, I. Reisinger, G. Logodi (Abt. Nuklearmesstechnik und Strahlenschutz (Prof. K. Jordan)) as well as the technical assistance of H. Dopslaff, F. Seipelt, H. Cordes and G. Baas are sincerely appreciated.

The reliable patience of K. Riensch who prepared and assembled the final manuscript as a CMS script file with continuous help from all the computer operators is particularly acknowledged.

Finally I am very much indebted to H. Langridge for his expertise in translation and for his critical control of my English.

D. P. P.

CONTENTS

1. INTRODUCTION

Over the last 20 years it is imaging that has become very important in Nuclear Medicine (2,157). Interest in the further development of non-imgaging techniques with single probes, which used to be employed exclusively before the invention of scanner and gamma camera, has receded into the background (36). In the case of computer-assisted dynamic scintigraphy, however, digital image sequences often only serve as aids for localizing ROIs (regions of interest) for the generation of time activity functions. The diagnostic interpretation of the study may take place less with the use of pictures than with the analysis of one-dimensional time-activity-histograms from ROIs. Signals of this kind can also often be obtained with much less effort and cost by means of single or multiple probes.

Activity distributions outside the field of view of a gamma-camera are completely ignored in routine investigations. As a result of the ubiquitous distribution of the radioindicator through the blood, on the other hand, a number of individual probes, which are attached to different parts of the body, can provide additional information in the fashion of special whole-body measurements.

The determination of glomerular filtration rates, of the subcutaneous resorption of radioactively labeled insulin, of the local Xe-133 clearance in the determination of blood flow, and of the I-123-(I-131) thyroid uptake, or hematological investigations with single probes are just a few examples which do not demand methods employing pictures (17,41,42,51,94,112,119,120,148,171,172). Other Nuclear Medicine procedures, such as, for example, radiocardiography, renography, lymphoscintigraphy, measurements of cerebrospinal fluid dynamics, or ferrokinetics require specialized expensive instrumentation within Nuclear Medicine departments with (large) stationary imaging equipment. The patient must remain under them without moving at all during the diagnostic examinations. Strict immobilisation during imaging procedures is a prerequisite for scintigraphy and functional imaging (Fig.1, left).

Procedures and investigations of this kind can be extended, completed or partially replaced by means of so-called storage-telemetric measurements with small detectors situated on or within the body of the patient (38-42,93,150,156,158,187). Small, battery-driven devices (e.g. mechanical or electronic memories) which the patient carries with him memorize the signals received from the nuclear radiation field by means of suitable sensors. So-called 'storage-telemetry' permits the carrying out of long-term measurements over hours, days and even longer periods. The patient retains his mobility. There are no restrictions to his movements. Measurements during sleep present no difficulties. Investigations on people under extreme working and environmental conditions, such as divers or pilots, are possible. Implantation of suitable nuclear radiation detectors, e.g. with injection needles, can be carried out (72,129,203,219).

A further clinical example of the desirable application of 'storage-telemetric' long-term measurements (with warning if values exceed boundary conditions) is the postoperative thrombosis surveillance of patients at risk by means of the radioiodinated fibrinogen-uptake-test (103,104,197,208). Nuclear Medicine measurements during surgery, in the case of invasive tests (e.g. catheterization), as well as in intensive care units are, in addition, of great interest and become a possible proposition.

In the case of 'storage-telemetric' signal registration, no data is transmitted through radio signals (182). Disturbances in electromagnetic wave propagation, and thus in the reception caused by electrical machinery, walls, shielded rooms e.g. operating rooms, cross-talk on several channels, great distances, change of position, therefore do not have to be taken into account. The nuclear radiation field, the carrier of the messages from inside the body, is registered in loco, in situ with detectors placed on the skin, introduced into body orifices or implanted (Fig. 1). It is memorized locally as a local countrate. The term 'telemetry' appears to be confusing for this. On the other hand, the term 'engymetry' proposed by PRETSCHNER (156,158) in 1980 (engys = nearby) makes clear the essential feature of measurements directly at the organ, independent of the position of the patient and without restricting his mobility (150,156,158). Non-imaging measurements near the organ concerned, without absorptive collimation, as in the case of the gamma camera, in addition permit a considerable reduction of the dose of the radioindicator. This means that the patient's exposure to radiation can be reduced.

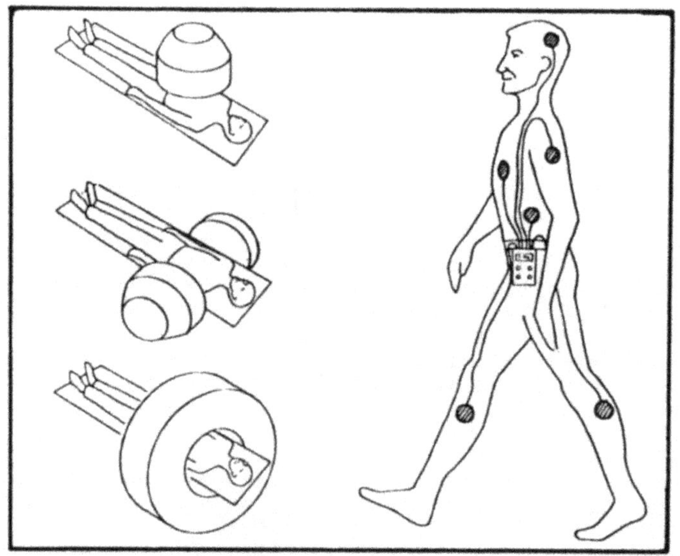

Fig. 1:
Non-imaging engymetry versus scintigraphy
Left: Conventional scintigraphy with stationary imaging equipment and necessary immobilization of the patient with temporally and locally restricted examinations
Right: Engymetry for Nuclear Medicine procedures, practically unrestricted in time and space

The use of radioindicators with longer effective half-life periods for the examination of slowly changing biomedical functions means that particularly low doses have to be applied for reasons of radiation safety. This results in low photon fluxes leading to bad statistics. Compensation is possible with loss of spatial resolution by local integration using large detector crystals. As the biomedical functions of interest change slowly (low frequency content), another trivial method of compensation is through long counting intervals. This is achieved by the use of small portable detectors fixed to or in the patient (Fig. 1). It is a characteristic feature of engymetry in Nuclear Medicine (156,158). Scintigrams are hardly possible in procedures of this kind because of low photon flux, nor are they necessary for many of the medical questions posed. A large number of pathophysiological functions have slow courses. One of the tasks of this book is to illustrate how such examinations could be made possible in registering and analysing slowly changing nuclear radiation fields emitted by patients, the radiant energy carrying pathophysiological messages.

This book is divided into three main sections. The first, SIGNAL REGISTRATION, deals with the detection of nuclear radiation emitted by the patient. Various engymetrically suitable radiation detectors were tested and developed specially for this purpose. After signal detection, a battery-powered electronic device, which can be programmed and which is carried by the patient, memorizes the measurement values simultaneously and continuously from four sensors. This device, patented in 1976 (161), was developed after the initial presentation of a prototype by PRÉTSCHNER and GETTNER (150).

In the second main section, INFORMATION PROCESSING, a concept of data handling for engymetric signals is developed with an inexpensive personal computer. An interactive analysis system with graphics for engymetric signals (DISYA) is described in the sense of 'alternative data processing' (179). It was programmed in ASSEMBLER, PASCAL and FORTRAN. Simple and complex mathematical analysis procedures for engymetric time-activity-histograms are available in DIALOG. Thus an inexpensive new tool was created. It was planned that this instrument should transfer the main work from the development of algorithmic means for solving problems by computer specialists ('solutions looking for problems' (155)) to non-algorithmic problem-solving by physicians (117). The clinical a priori knowledge which the doctor as a non-specialist in computer techniques has is to be employed in an optimum way (92). Thus procedures which are already known can probably be employed more effectively within the framework of engymetry.

The analysis of the novel engymetric time sequences which is in each case clinically most appropriate has not been sufficiently tested for a number of fields of medical application, or is even to a large extent unknown. The goal was to make problem-solving easier for the scientist on the basis of a comprehensive program library of algorithms which have proved their worth in Nuclear Medicine, and of neutral mathematical methods of analysis, as, for example, from compartment analysis (linear system theory) (73,96,122,183,214,215).

The third main section deals with CLINICAL APPLICATIONS and the clinical results of engymetry in Nuclear Medicine in different fields of application with engygrams from more than 400 patients. The fields of application of procedures which have proved their worth in Nuclear Medicine are extended by the new portable devices and by the wide range of analytical possibilities with graphical support in dialog with the personal computer system. In addition, new questions are raised concerning clinical areas and experimental research in which the imaging procedures of Nuclear Medicine cannot at present be made available, or only made available by considerably more expensive means.

The engymetric system described in this book has been clinically tested and proved for more than two years. Experience with individual preliminary steps in the sytem has existed since 1975.

2. SIGNAL REGISTRATION

A signal is 'the time course of a physical magnitude which transmits a message (and thus reproduces information)' (29). The physical magnitude is the material or energy carrier of the message. Information is produced after appropriate preprocessing of the signals and interpretation of the messages by a human receiver. His ability to subjectively realize abstract and theoretical model concepts determines the interpretation of objective signals. Interpretations usually change during the process of obtaining scientific knowledge.

The physical magnitude as the carrier of the diagnostic message in Nuclear Medicine (NM) is a nuclear radiation field. It is variable in time, space and energy. It is emitted by the patient following incorporation and distribution of artificial radionuclides. After its detection with one of the common imaging devices used in NM (scanner, gamma camera), a projective representation of the radiation field is generally produced as a series of two-dimensional scintigrams p(x,y,t), which the physician interprets (157).

In the case of signal registration with single probes the dependence of the signal on spatial variables (x,y) is usually not explicitly stated. It is regarded as one-dimensional. The essential anatomical information, however, is retained through the fixed and known position of the detectors on or within the body.

The local nuclear radiation field is converted into an impulse rate.

$$N(t)=\int_{-x}^{x}\int_{-y}^{y}\int_{0}^{z} e\left(\sqrt{\xi^2+\eta^2},\ \zeta\right)\ c\ (\xi,\eta,\zeta,t)\ d\xi\ d\eta\ d\zeta \qquad (2.1)$$

c(x,y,z,t) is the time-dependent concentration of the radioindicator within the field of view of the detector. e(x,y,z) describes the (time-constant) detection efficiency dependent on the position and on the photon energy of the source with the inclusion of absorption and scatter. Equation (2.1) is valid after BASSINGTHWAIGHTE (18) for axially symmetrical isocount curves of the detector, with x,y as the distance from the axis of symmetry and z as the depth from the photon absorption layer of the detector.

The non-separable superposition of radiation from various depths of the body, absorption, scatter, additional background radiation and the depth-dependence of the transfer function of the detector system lead to serious distortions with regard to the linear relationship between registered countrate and activity concentration in the volume of interest. Apart from computerized emission tomography these effects can in individual cases be compensated for by means of models through the inclusion of a priori information (153,154,157). According to eq.2.1, in the case of engymetric measurements activities in the immediate vicinity of the detector are particularly well detected. On the one hand this makes it difficult for quantitative measurements of nuclear radiation to be made from more distantly situated tissue volumes. But on the other hand it is very advantageous for close-range measurements (engymetric auto-collimation).

The engymetric system for signal registration and analysis, MIESSY (Medical Information Extraction and Storage SYstem), consists of three subsystems (Fig. 2.1) for:

1. radiation detection
2. primary storage of signals
3. secondary storage, analysis, and display of data (158).

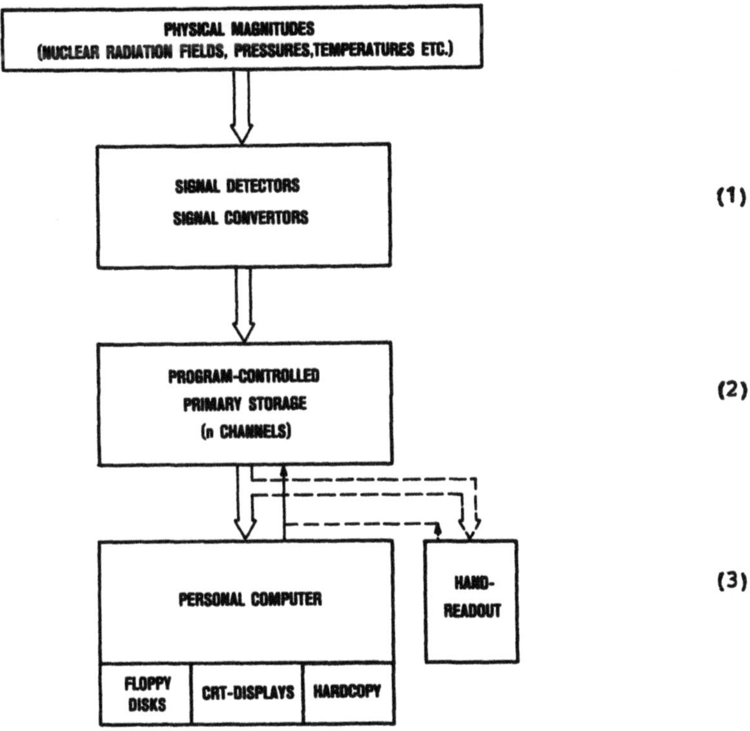

Fig. 2.1:
Diagram of MIESSY (Medical Information Extraction and Storage SYstem) with three subsystems for radiation detection (1), primary storage (2), secondary storage and signal analysis (3).

2.1 Radiation Detection

Miniaturised GM-counter tubes, scintillation and semiconductor detectors are suitable as portable, battery-powered detectors (39,51,68,88,89,90,100,129,150,158,199,219). In the case of most applications discussed here, energy selective counting is at first not the main point of interest. Pure counter operation without a pulse-height analyser, as in the case of GM-counters and silicon avalanche detectors, is sufficient. At present CdTe (Z=40.5) and HgI_2 (Z=80.5) seem to be the most suitable of the solid-state detectors for use at room temperature (88,89,90,129,163,174,185,219). They show good energy discrimination, relatively high detection efficiency and miniaturisation. They do, however, demand charge amplifiers and special casings which protect against microphony (30). This is especially important with medical measurements on out-patients. Their detection efficiency greatly decreases with higher energies (>200 keV). Silicon avalanche detectors and drifted Si(Li)diodes, which can also be easily miniaturised, are particularly suitable as engymetric detectors

(72,100,199). Some promising experience has already been gained with these (8,100,199). NaI(Tl) and $Bi_4Ge_3O_{12}$ (abbrev.: BGO) can also be considered as portable scintillators[3] with battery-driven miniature photomultiplier tubes (PMT) in the higher energy range. A detector unit with PMT and battery-powered electronics, however, cannot be miniaturised so easily, and consumes more current than semiconductor detectors (Fig.2.2,D, Fig.2.12). Problems of detection and measurement of nuclear radiation in Nuclear Medicine are treated by ROLLO (169), SORENSON and PHELPS (188), and JORDAN (99).

Fig. 2.2 shows a collection of engymetric radiation detectors as well as the portable program-controlled primary storage module.

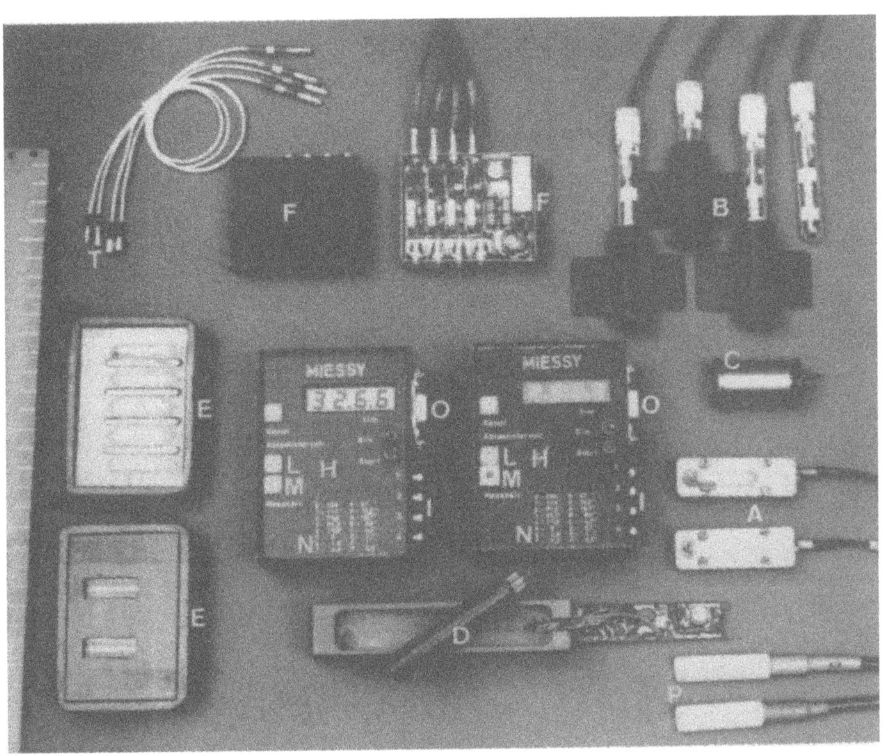

Fig. 2.2:
Radiation detectors and primary signal storage modules (scale in cm).

A: 2 GM tubes with brass collimators
B: 4 GM tubes in acrylic glass, over which slotted lead tubes can be slid for collimation
C: GM counter with larger counting volume
D: BGO detector with miniature PMT and associated electronics
E: 2 arrangements for double nuclide measurements, consisting of 2 GM counters for low and high energies visible in the window, and 3 GM counters only for high energies under a lead cover
F: 2 high-voltage generators and amplifiers, each for 4 channels, closed on the left and open on the right. Upper 4 connections for detectors, lower ones for storage unit
H: 2 storage units with 4 inputs (I) and output (O) for readout
L: revolving switch for 16-fold adjustable sampling intervals t_s
M: revolving switch for 16-fold adjustable integration periods t_c
N: Table with sampling and counting intervals on top of primary storage unit (Table 2.1)
T: CdTe - detectors
P: 2 Silicon solid state avalanche radiation detectors

2.1.1 GEIGER-MÜLLER COUNTERS, COLLIMATORS

Gas-filled, self-quenching GM counter tubes have low detection efficiency and counting rate limitations (99). However, they can be delivered quickly, are reliable and not expensive (39,150,158,218). The incapsulating of GM counter tubes in suitable synthetics or their inclusion in small, mechanically stable synthetic tubes (Fig. 2.2,B) has proved to be satisfactory for measurements on the patient even without special collimation because of the inherent autocollimation of small absorption volumes. Non-collimated detectors have to be attached to parts of the body which are subjected to as little irradiation as possible from other parts of the body, such as moved extremities, filling urinary bladder etc.

The following examples of clinical applications in section 4 illustrate GM counters employed in various arrangements (218). The self-quenching VALVO Type ZP 1320 (filled with Ne, Ar, Halogen) can be included in casings of brass or lead which serve as the collimator (Fig. 2.2,A,B) (218). Several collimated individual detectors are attached to the cuff of a sphygmomanometer for areal measurements (Fig. 2.3). The characteristics of an individual probe collimated with brass after Fig. 2.2,A are shown in Fig. 2.4 for two energy ranges (Tc-99m: 140 keV, I-131: 365 keV). Another type of collimator consists of a slotted lead tube which can be slid over the GM detector (Fig. 2.2,B). A special stiffening plate prevents turning in the longitudinal axis.

Above counting rates of 10,000 cpm counting losses can exceed 1%.

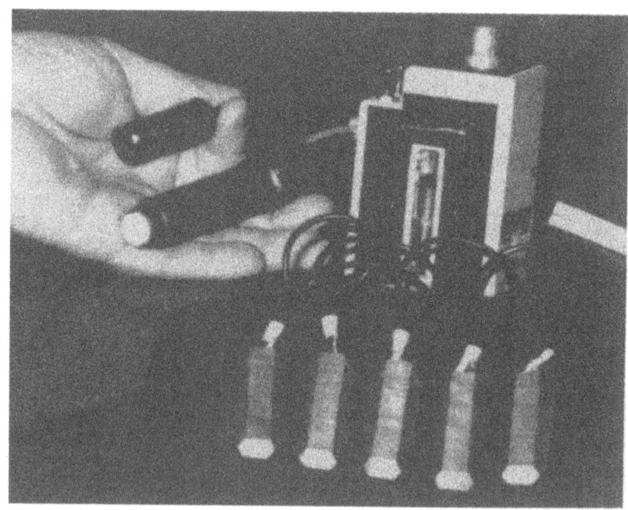

Fig. 2.3:
Nuclear radiation detectors
Above left: miniature GM counter tube, below it a 12 mm BGO crystal with miniature photomultiplier
Centre: storage apparatus with integrated GM counter tube (as in Fig. 2.5).
Below: 5 GM counter tubes with brass collimators attached to the cuff of a sphygmomanometer

The GM counters are operated at 600 V, generated by a battery-powered high-voltage supply with a miniature transformer (Fig. 2.2,F). The high impedance and lack of reference of the portable battery-powered high-voltage generator to the earth potential guarantee protection of the patient in the case of possible short-circuiting of the GM detectors.

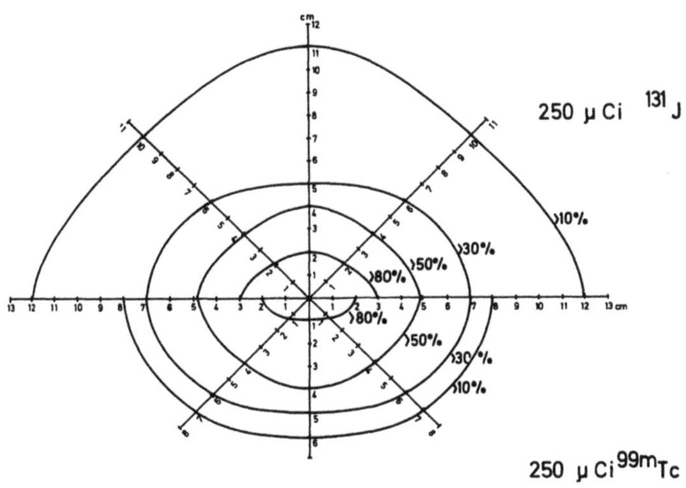

Fig. 2.4:
Isoimpulse curves of a point source at a distance of 5 cm (air) with a variable distance to the central point of an individual detector collimated with brass after Fig. 2.2,A

During the developmental stages of MIESSY a battery powered radiation detection and display unit shown in Fig. 2.5 was constructed in 1975. It consists of a built-in GM-counter tube, a high voltage generator, and a scaler-timer. The number of photons recorded, as well as the counting interval, are displayed on the LCD. This device was used for thrombosis detection with the radiofibrinogen uptake test after aorto-coronary venous bypass surgery for treatment of coronary heart disease (section 4.1) and for detection of right-to-left shunts in children (section 4.2.1).

Continuous storage of countrates from radiation detectors as with the primary storage module of section 2.2 is not possible with this unit. Nevertheless it has proved very useful for initial and quick orientation about unknown nuclear radiation fields. Apart from its proven usefulness in thrombosis detection the instrument allows immediate diagnosis of flow stops in cerebrospinal fluid shunts (section 4.6.1).

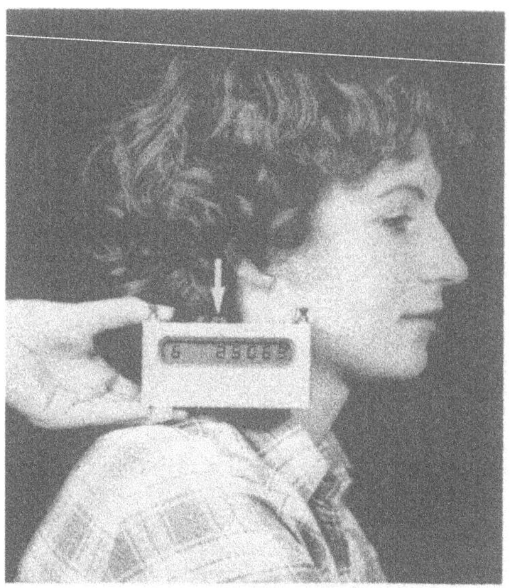

Fig. 2.5:
Battery-powered scaler-timer with liquid crystal display (LCD) in front and built-in GM counter tube on the rear side, as in Fig. 2.3. Switches for different counting intervals of the timer (arrow). On the display to the left the coded counting interval (6:2^6 sec = 64 sec), to the right the number of detected events during the counting interval

Dual Radioisotope Counting

Fig. 2.7 shows another type of detector with 10 GM counter tubes. There are two layers, each consisting of 5 embedded in acrylic glass lying next to each other. A lead slide of variable thickness can separate the two detector layers, so that two radionuclides with different energies can be measured simultaneously. In order to demonstrate the separation of scatter, Fig. 4.4 shows two radiocardiography curves registered by this detector unit after i.v. injection of 4 mCi H_2O-15. The larger curve was measured in front of, and the smaller one behind, the 4 mm thick lead slide. A further detector arrangement suitable for double radionuclide measurements is shown in Figs. 2.2,E, 2.8. Here the GM counters do not lie on top of each other, as in Fig. 2.7, but beside each other, separated by brass. In clinical application the GM dual radioisotope detectors are used for measurements in chronic venous insufficiency (section 4.3). Br-82 is used to label the extracellular compartment. The intravascular space is distinguished with in vivo labeled red blood cells using Tc-99m (158).

Two channels are provided for with the arrangement of the GM-tubes in Fig. 2.8. Two counters seen in the lead windows are connected for channel 1. Three GM-tubes placed behind 4 mm thick lead shielding are connected for channel 2.

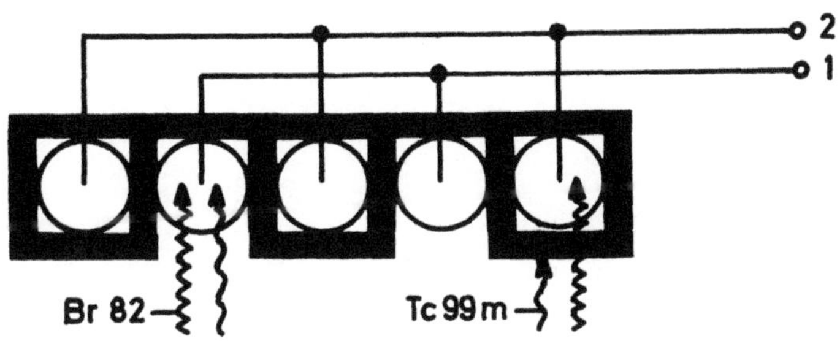

Fig. 2.6:
Dual radionuclide counting. Br-82 photons penetrate lead, Tc-99m ones do not. Circles: GM-counter tubes

Counts C_{1Br} in channel 1 without and C_{2Br} in channel 2 with the lead filter plates are given by a standard sample of Br-82 only. The ratio of counts is

$$r = \frac{c_{1Br}}{c_{2Br}} \tag{2.2}$$

A sample of Tc-99m gives counts C_{1Tc} only in channel 1 because most Tc-99m 140 keV photons cannot penetrate the 4 mm lead filter. Counts C_1 in channel 1 and C_2 in channel 2 are measured from a mixture with both Br-82 and Tc-99m.

$$c_1 = c_{1Br} + c_{1Tc} \tag{2.3}$$

$$c_2 = c_{2Br} \tag{2.4}$$

With r from the Br-82 standard sample, counts C_{1Tc} in channel 1 for Tc-99m only are for dual-radioisotope counting

$$c_{1Tc} = c_1 - c_2 \cdot r \tag{2.5}$$

When mixtures of two other different radionuclides are used, similar relationships also hold. They become more complicated if the lower energy radioisotope should contribute essentially to the counts in the lead-filtered high energy channel.

In addition, deviations from linear relationships between tissue concentrations of radiolabels and countrates exist because of measurement geometry regarding the two unshielded detectors for channel 1 and the three detectors for the high energy channel 2. Furthermore, backscatter is not taken into account at all.

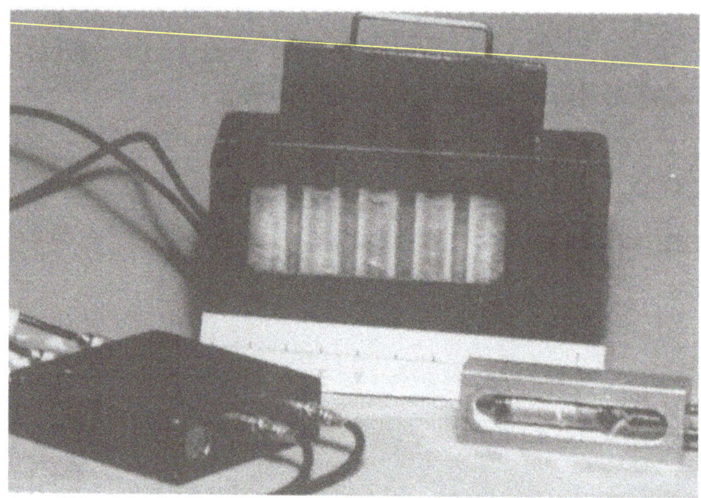

Fig. 2.7:
Arrangement for double radionuclide measurements
Left: high-voltage generator (600 V/channel) and amplifier for 2 channels
Centre: 10 GM counter tubes in two layers separable by lead slides. The window shows the 5 front counter tubes embedded in acrylic glass
Right: Single GM counter tube in brass collimator. Scale in cm

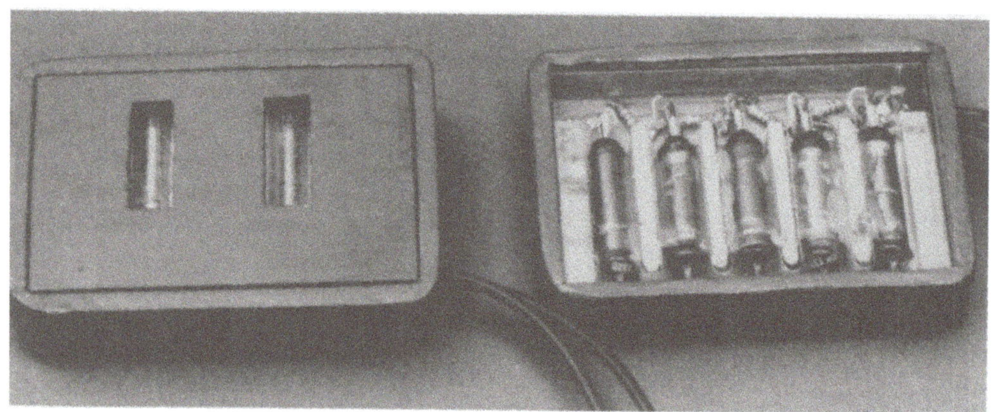

Fig. 2.8:
GM detector for double radionuclide measurement.
Left: closed, two GM counters in the window for channel 1
Right: open, three GM counters behind lead plate for channel 2

2.1.2 SEMICONDUCTOR DETECTORS

MARTINI (129), WALFORD et al. (203) and VOGEL (199) provide a review of the state of technology in the employment of solid-state detectors in Nuclear Medicine and radiobiology.

Fig. 2.9 shows 4 CdTe semiconductor detectors, each with a diameter of 3 and 5 mm, produced by Radiation Monitoring Devices. Inc., Watertown MA 02172. For their protection and sterilisation they are slid into specially produced acrylic glass tubes, as shown in Fig. 2.9. The acrylic glass block of Fig. 2.10 can accommodate 4 detectors, and, for example, in the case of neurosurgical operations they can be placed on the open brain tissues to measure local blood flow. Intraoperative measurements of myocardial circulation before and after aortocoronary venous bypass surgery are also possible. Charge preamplifier, subsequent amplifier and bias voltage unit are powered by batteries that can be recharged. Special collimation is possible. Fig. 2.11 shows an arrangement for the measuring of flow in a catheter which is intended for ventriculoatrial or ventriculoperitoneal shunts in disorders of cerebrospinal fluid dynamics (see Section 4.6.1).

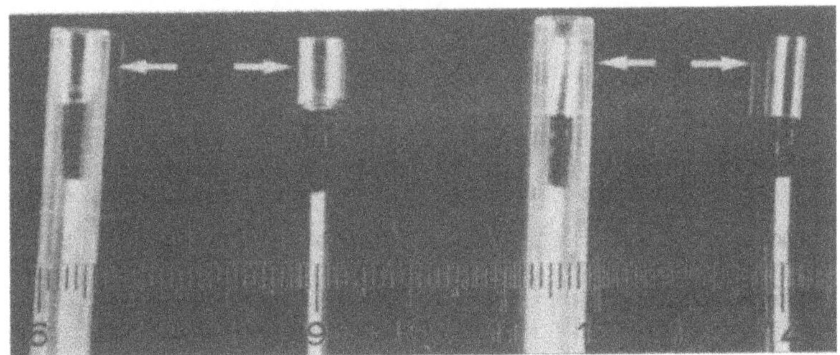

Fig. 2.9:
Four miniaturised CdTe detectors (arrows) without collimator. Two of them in acrylic glass tubes

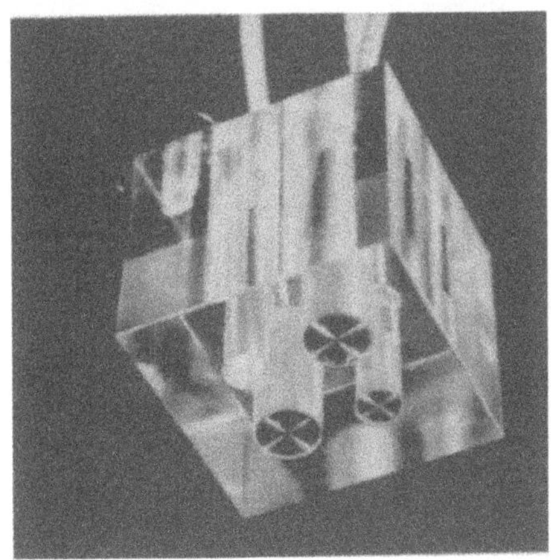

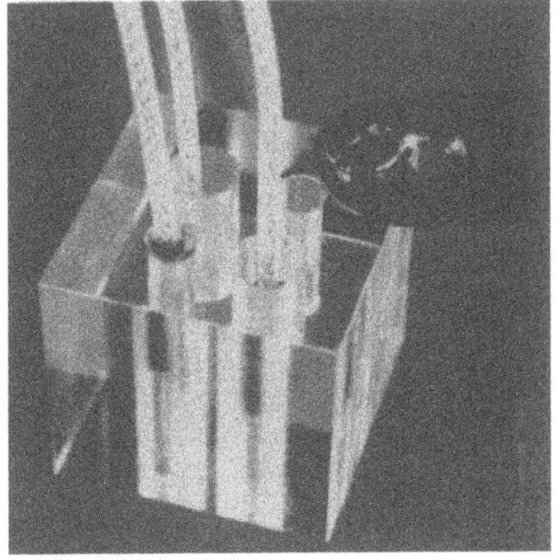

Fig. 2.10:
Acrylic glass block with holder and three embedded CdTe detectors for intraoperative measurements (two views)

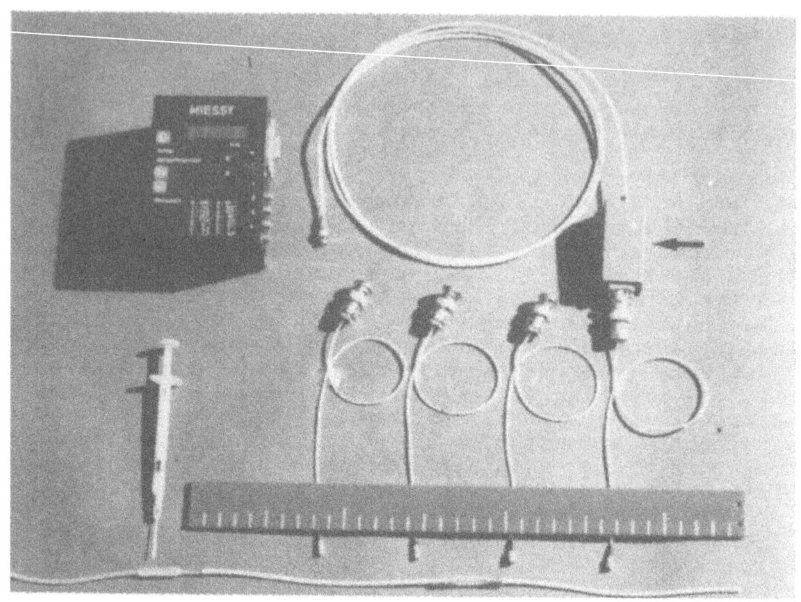

Fig. 2.11:
Scheme of the arrangement for a shunt flow measurement with four CdTe detectors. Attached charge amplifier (arrow). Storage unit top left

Fig. 2.12 shows HgI_2 detectors. They were made available by H.SCHOLZ (163,178), Philips Research Laboratory, Aachen. These detectors are being tested.

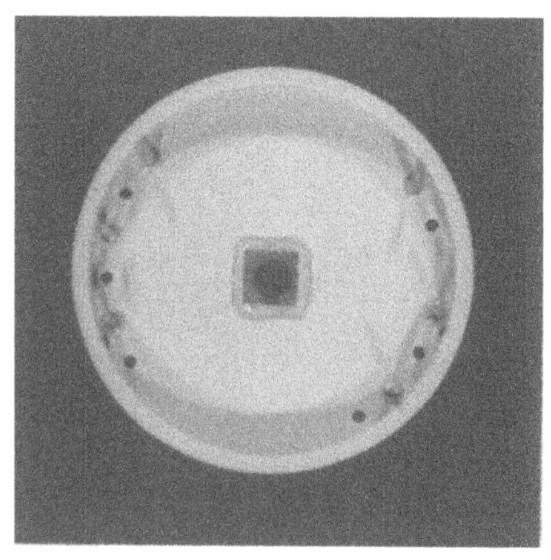

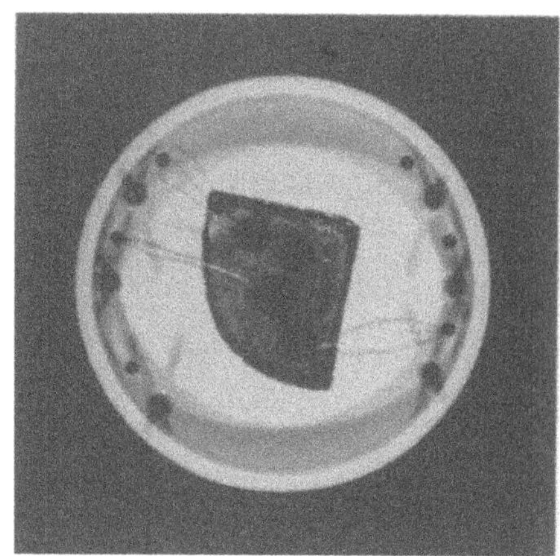

Fig. 2.12:
HgI_2 detectors with opened housing
Left : a small individual detector
Right: a large crystal with three-fold contacting to increase efficiency

HASSAN et al. (89,90) describe a 'radio-pill' that can be swallowed, the HgI_2 detector of which is described as being suitable for the application of Tc-99m and P-32.

Silicon avalanche detectors (Figs. 2.2,P, 2.13) and Si(Li) diodes (100,199) are particularly suitable for the detection of charged particles (Fig. 2.13, Avalanche Nuclear Inc., Calif. 92649).

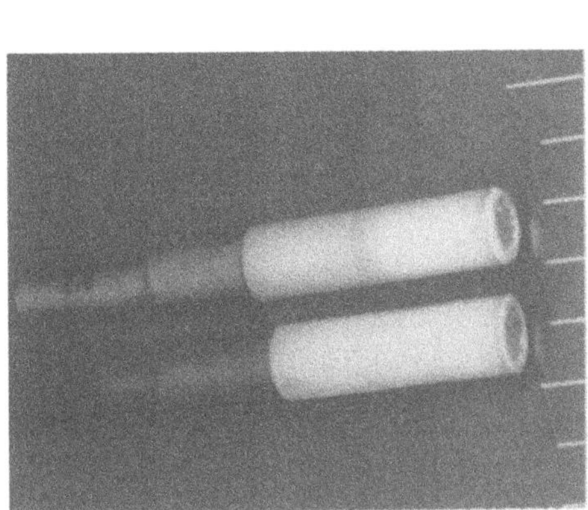

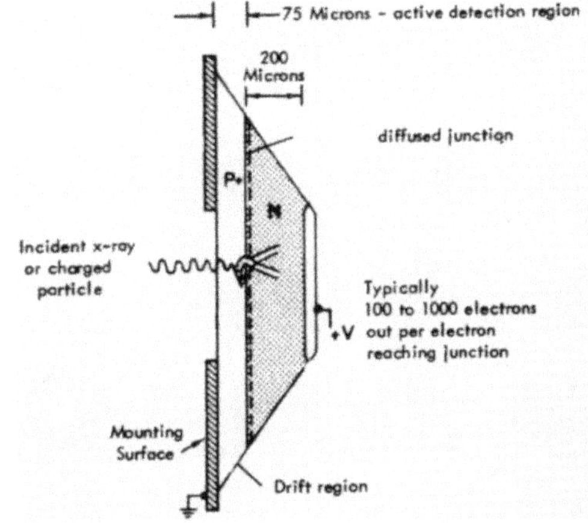

Fig. 2.13:
Two silicon avalanche detectors (Fig. 2.2,P), with scheme (right)

So far we do not have sufficient clinical experience with these. KARLSBERG et al. (100) report on good results with blood flow measurements on the myocardium in animal experiments.

Thermoluminescence dosimeters, which have to be replaced every two hours, have also been used according to BOJSEN et al. (37).

2.1.3 SCINTILLATION DETECTORS

Because of the availability of the 'physiologically' interesting positron emitters C-11, N-13, O-15 through the department's own cyclotron, measurements at higher energies are of particular interest. NaI(Tl), otherwise the standard scintillator in diagnostic measurements in Nuclear Medicine, is less suitable with higher photon energies. Bismuth-germanate, $Bi_4Ge_3O_{12}$, is being used increasingly for measurements of positron annihilation radiation (7,35) as a non-hygroscopic, inert scintillator with rather high mass number and density. Miniaturisation and battery operation cannot be achieved so easily because of the necessary PMT with relatively high current consumption. Figs. 2.2,D, 2.3 show a miniaturised unit with PMT .

For measurements of radioelements with emission of high energies the Harshaw Chemical Company specially produced 2 BGO integral line detectors with an 8 mm radial boring (Fig. 2.14). Detailed specifications are to be found in the data sheets (35). Catheters can be slid through the boring, the activity content of which (liquid, gaseous) can be measured with great accuracy. Fig. 2.15 shows time-activity-histograms after bolus injection of 1 µCi/50 µl $(C\text{-}11)O_3^{2-}$ in one catheter with a flow of 4 µl/min. This unit cannot be carried by the patient. It is intended for flow measurements, e.g. in the heart catheter laboratory, during operations and for research. Its connection with MIESSY lies in the simple inexpensive way of collecting, storing and analysing data.

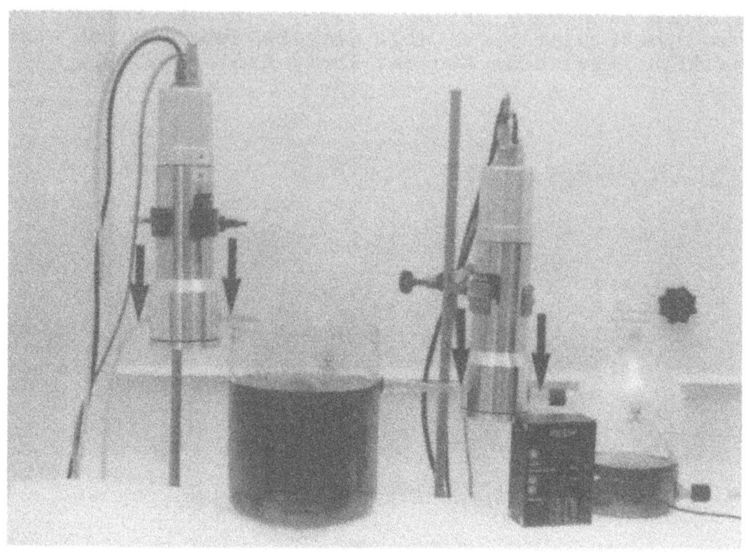

Fig. 2.14:
Two bored-through BGO detectors with catheters pushed through (arrows). Realized model of Fig. 3.26. Primary storage unit below right

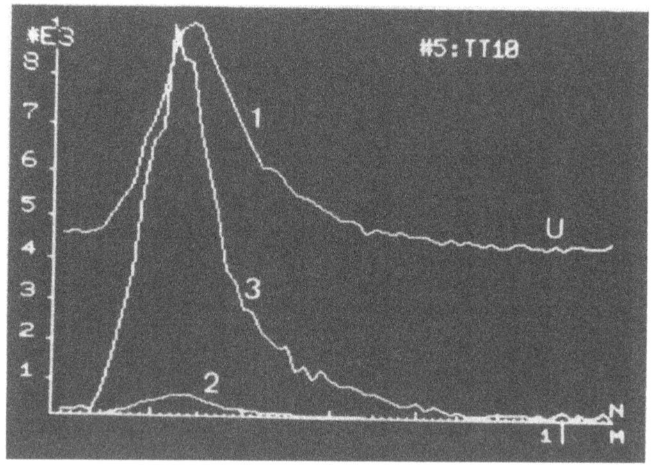

Fig. 2.15:
Bolus flow (40 µl/min) of 1 µCi/50µl (C-11)O_3^{2-} through BGO detectors after Fig. 2.14. Discrimination of a constant background U (1) through raising of the threshold (2). (3): normalization of (2) to max. of (1) with DISYA.
Sampling interval: 1 sec, counting interval: 0.5 sec, total measurement time: 64 sec. Abscissa in min (M)

In the case of measurements with positron emitters there remains the basic problem of the high penetrability of photons after annihilation (511 keV). Shielding or collimation of the detectors necessary for this is too bulky for portable probes (for measurement tasks using the bored BGO crystals (Fig. 2.14)). The absorptive shielding can be neglected for measurement tasks using the bored BGO crystals if one filters the detected photon energies electronically.

With a single probe, only one of the two simultaneously, but diametrically emitted gamma photons is picked up by the detector after annihilation. If, however, the radiation source is situated within the detector (catheter pushed through, Fig. 2.14), then both quanta can be detected in coincidence. Scattering photons from outside are rejected through the appropriate choice of the discriminator threshold.

As an example of this measurement technique Fig. 2.15 shows the bolus flow already mentioned of 1 µCi/50 µl $(C\text{-}11)O_3^{2-}$ through the BGO detector according to Fig. 2.14. Curve 1 contains the constant background radiation U. In curve 2 under the same test conditions the background radiation is limited electronically, while the discriminator threshold is raised >511 keV. Curve 3 is displayed after normalization of curve 2 to the maximum of curve 1 by using DISYA.

2.2 Primary Storage of Signals

The signals produced by the first subsystem (radiation detection) are transferred to the storage device separately for each channel and fed into an impulse counter with 5 decades (binary coded decimal (BCD)). The lower 4 decades can be represented decimally at the same time by means of a liquid crystal display. In addition to the display of the real-time countrates of the selected channel, the actual status of the primary storage subsystem is indicated by different signs. For example, counting is indicated by a flickering colon, or the end of measurement by a dot.

The counter content is fed into the memory after the end of each counting interval. The next counting interval is started after each new sampling interval. It can be preselected in the same way as the counting period. The maximum countrate is 1 MHz/channel.

If overflow of the counter decades should occur, with the result that they are reset to zero and started again, this can be corrected by the software of the third subsystem.

Fig. 2.16 shows the block diagram of a program-controlled four-channel device for primary data storage. Several microprograms exist for various functions such as signal storing, reading, or testing of the equipment. Fig. 2.17 shows flow charts of two such programs for data input and output. Program and data memories can be extended independently. The integrated circuits used correspond to military requirements and specifications. They are especially suitable for employment in nuclear radiation fields, e.g. in space research (198).

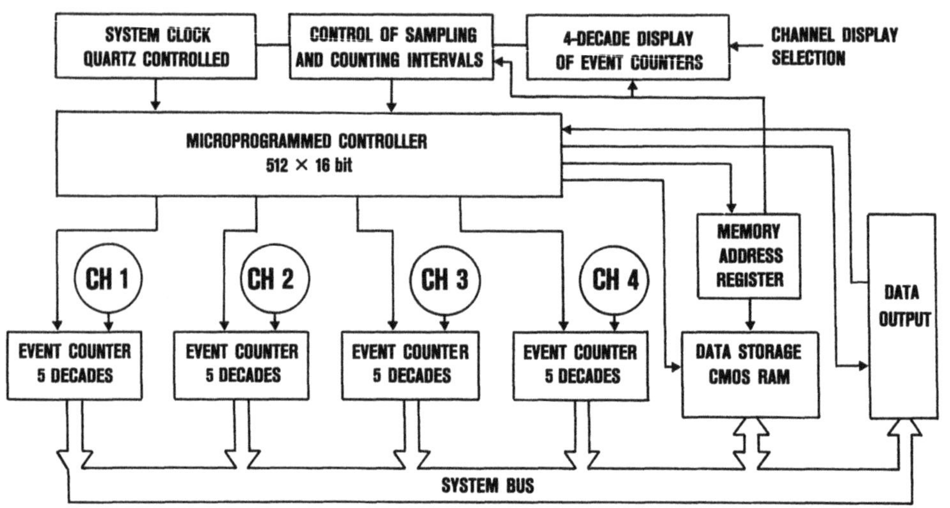

Fig. 2.16:
Block circuit diagram of a primary 4-channel storage device. 4 detector inputs CH1 - CH4

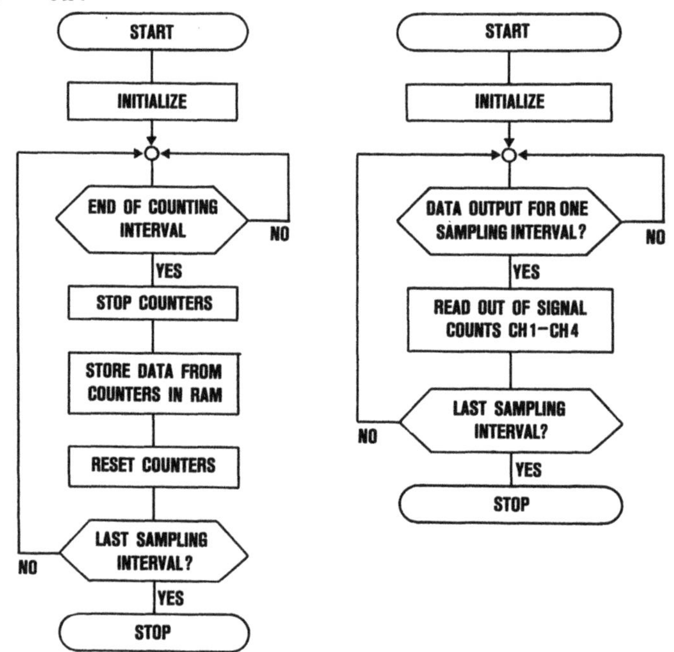

Fig. 2.17:
Flow charts of two programs in the portable storage device for data storing (left) and reading (right)

In the case of the unit shown in Figs. 2.2,H, 2.21 counting and sampling periods can be programmed independently of each other in 16 steps from 0.25 sec to 5 hours through a crystal-controlled time base (4 MHz) (Fig. 2.2,L,M).

Two switches, S_c and S_s, control data collection by means of two parameters, t_c and t_s, the counting and sampling intervals being identical for all 4 channels. Each switch has 16 positions. Both switch positions, S_c for t_c and S_s for t_s, can be combined with condition

$$S_s \geq S_c \tag{2.6}$$

If one chooses switch position $S_s = 2$, for example, then 14 positions 2-F are possible for S_c (table 2.1). 64 single function values can be stored for each channel. Total measurement time T_N for all channels, therefore, is $T_N = 64t_s$. The longest time T_N for one continuous measurement is about 12.5 days, the shortest about 32 sec. Table 2.1 and Fig. 2.18 show all the data collection parameters as well as their time relationships.

Switch-positions (S_s, S_c)	Sampling interval t_s		Counting interval t_c	
	min	sec	min	sec
0	285	52	142	56
1	142	56	71	28
2	71	28	35	44
3	35	44	17	52
4	17	52	8	56
5	8	56	4	28
6	4	28	2	14
7	2	14	1	7
8	1	7		33.5
9		33.5		16.75
A		16.75		8.38
B		8.38		4.19
C		4.19		2.08
D		2.08		1.05
E		1.05		0.52
F		0.52		0.26

Table 2.1:
Sampling intervals t_s and counting intervals t_c

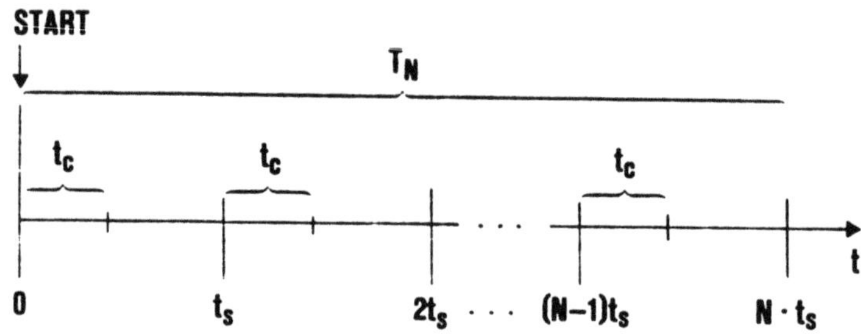

Fig. 2.18:
Time relationships for signal collection with primary storage module
T_N total measurement time
t_c counting interval
t_s sampling interval

Detected photons of the radiation field being measured are counted during integration interval t_c in Fig. 2.18. Changes in countrate during t_c cannot be detected. For the construction of time-activity histograms the n-th result of integrating counts during t_c is estimated to be in the middle of the counting interval t_c. For time value t_n of the n-th integration over t_c

$$t_n = \frac{t_C}{2} + (n-1)\ t_s \ ; \quad 1 < n < N \qquad (2.7)$$

Small hardware changes in the primary storage module lead to other tables of t_c and t_s resulting, for example, in longer total measurement periods T_N.

When a measurement is being set up, the positions of switches S_c and S_s have to be carefully matched to the given dose of radioindicator with regard to

1.) counting statistics
2.) sampling theorem (the signal can be exactly reconstructed if sampled at least at double the rate of the highest signal frequency component).

In practical routine it is advisable to make several measurements on long processes with separate readouts of data, each morning for example. This simplifies the control of the whole measurement procedure, especially regarding the correct position of the radiation detectors. These are easily misplaced in the clinical environment.

As an indication of the long-term constancy of MIESSY, Fig. 2.19 shows the example of a measurement over 200 days via one channel with a GM counter with constant measurement geometry and one set of batteries for high voltage, amplifier and primary storage unit. The tabulated value of the physical half-life of Co-57 is 330 days (181).

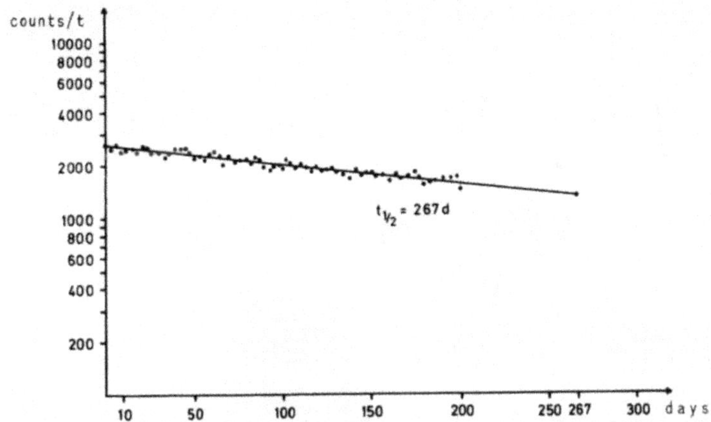

Fig. 2.19:
Long-term constancy measurement over 200 days with one set of batteries. Source: 500 µCi Co-57 in air

2.3 Reading, Secondary Storing, Analysis and Display of Signals

The third subsystem serves signal reading, secondary storing, display and further processing of the primarily stored measurement values (countrates) during and after completion of the test. It exists in two forms:

- portable, battery-powered hand signal reading unit (Fig. 2.20)
- personal computer system (Fig. 2.21)

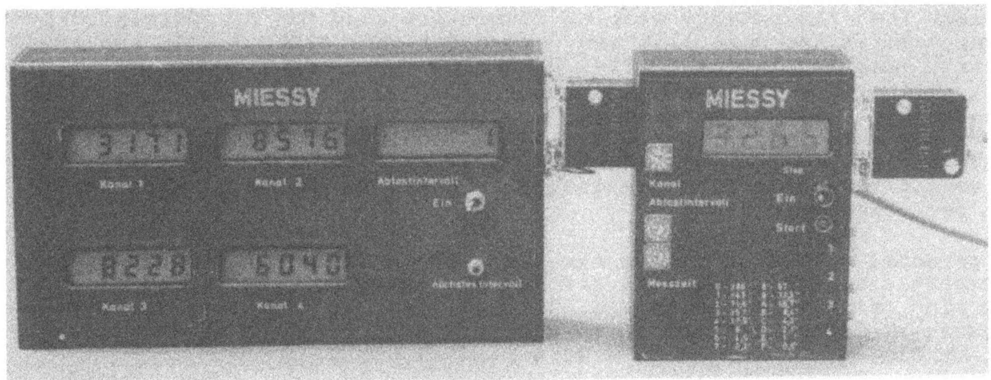

Fig 2.20:
Storing unit (right) with attached signal hand reading unit (left). As an example, the first measurement values of 4 stored time-activity-histograms are displayed

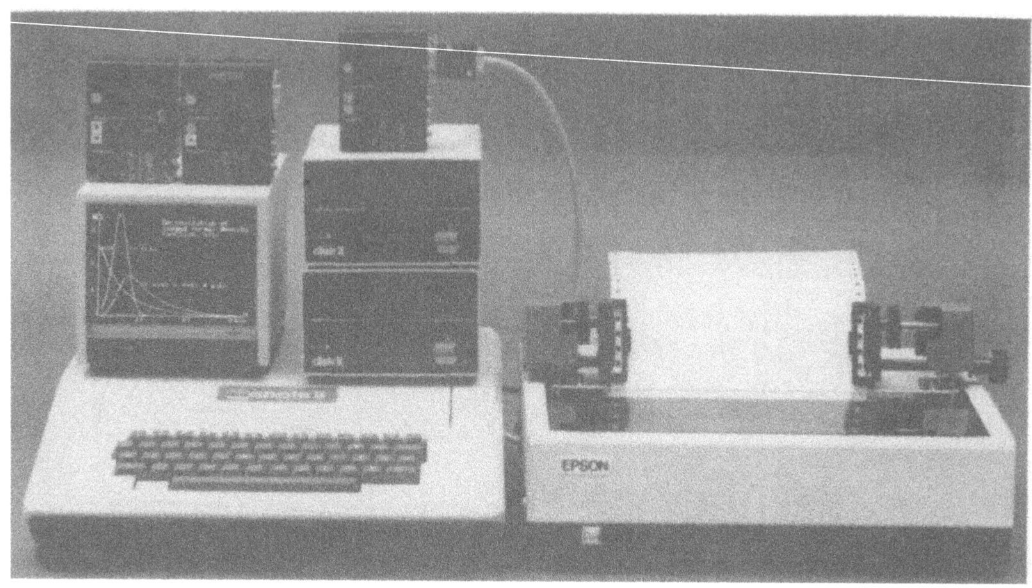

Fig. 2.21:
Analysis, display and secondary storing system.
The following are standing on top of the microcomputer (APPLE II):
left : videomonitor, and above two storing devices
middle: two diskette drive assemblies with storing device on top, connected for readout
right : printer
On the monitor: the time-activity-histograms of Fig. 3.30

In the case of the portable signal hand reading unit, the measurement values from the primary storing device are read out by pressing a button, and at the same time are shown for each channel with the appropriate sampling interval (Fig. 2.20).

Reading out data in such a way is time-consuming. Nevertheless, the portable reading out unit is inexpensive and particularly useful for testing purposes. Graphical display and further analysis of the time-activity-histograms, manually read out number by number, have to be performed separately.

A personal computer system has been chosen (Fig. 2.21) to combine automatic readout, display and further analysis. Using the same connecting cable as shown in Fig. 2.20 all data (4 time series) from subsystem II are transferred to the personal computer system during a short dialog session (Fig. 2.22).

```
EXECUTE WHAT FILE? E1
FILENAME?-->             #5:ENGYGRAM019
PAT.NAME?-->             PETER P. MED.HOCHSCHULE HANNOVER, 01051900, DEPARTMENT I
DATUM?-->                1-MAY-1982
NUKLID?VERBINDUNG?-->IN-111 OXINE PLATELETS, 1.5 MCI, 81 KG, 1.78 M
ABTASTINTERVALL?-->      6
MESSZEIT?-->             6
KOMMENTAR?-->            1 COR 2 SPLEEN 3 LIVER 4 HEAD 5 KIDNEY R 6 KIDNEY L 7 LEG L
     CONNECT MISSY
  DRUECKE STARTTASTE
TIPPE ZAHL
```

Fig. 2.22:
Example of a data collection dialog before transfer of stored data from subsystem II on to a diskette of the personal computer system.

E1	Name of executable PASCAL host program for reading data from primary storage unit
FILENAME?-->	Volume # of output device (diskette: #5:) and filename ENGYGRAM019 as identifier of all information stored on the diskette for this particular patient
PAT.NAME?-->	patient name, identification, doctor, etc.
DATUM?-->	date of reading in data from primary storage unit
NUKLID?VERBINDUNG?-->	radionuclide, chemical compound, dose injected
ABTASTINTERVALL?-->	sampling interval t_s (Fig. 2.18)
MESSZEIT?-->	counting interval t_c (Fig. 2.18)
KOMMENTAR?-->	free comment, here, for example, numbering of detectors, the first lying over the heart, the sixth over the left kidney
CONNECT MISSY	with connection cable
DRUECKE STARTTASTE	starts program 2 (Fig. 2.17) in primary storage unit
TIPPE ZAHL	press key of any number; starts EXTERNAL assembly routine in PASCAL host program E1

A PASCAL host program with a separately assembled assembly-language EXTERNAL procedure (15) reads the four time series into a file and record structure (Figs. 3.9, 3.10). It contains information on patient, measurement, radionuclide type and dosage, as well as free comment, asked for interactively during dialog. Fig. 3.9 shows the file and record structure as one variable PATIENT declared in the PASCAL program.

The actual transfer of data after the end of the dialog asking for patient and measurement specific information takes 750 msec. Only for this time is subsystem II connected to subsystem III.

One diskette file with the original data of one patient measurement uses 3 blocks. One side of a diskette with 35 tracks, each divided into 16 sectors, contains 280 blocks. Because of the directory, using blocks 2-5, which may store information for up to 77 different files, one diskette using both sides can hold original engymetric information from 2*77 = 154 patients.

2.4 Quality Control

A special test device has been developed for the quality maintenance and quality control of MIESSY. It consists of a lead container, into which 8 GM counter tubes are slid radially from outside as far as the stop (Fig. 2.23). A syringe with a defined radioactivity is introduced from above. This guarantees the substantial constancy of the measurement conditions, especially with regard to the measurement geometry. The 8 GM counters are attached to two storing devices.

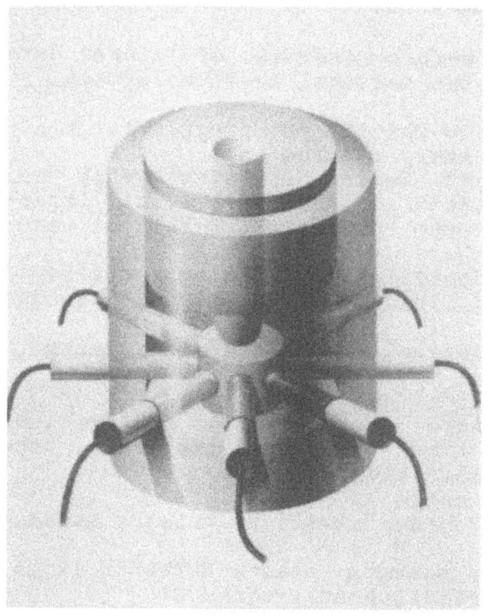

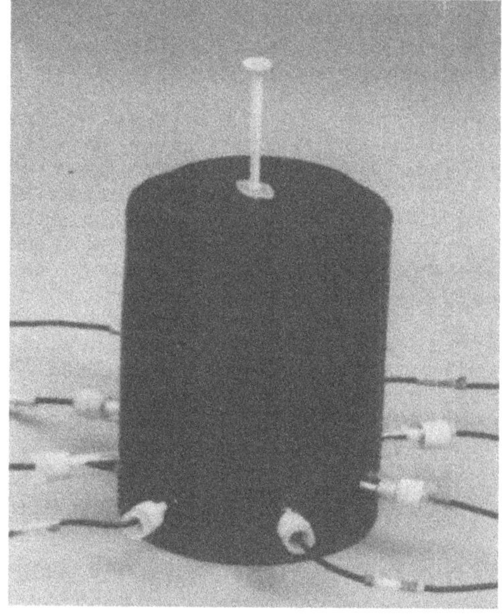

Fig. 2.23:
Test device for the quality control of MIESSY. The model shows 7 of the 8 GM counter tubes pushed in as far as the stop. The upper slid-in unit shows the apparatus for receiving the radioactivity
Right: the completed apparatus after the model with GM counters and syringe with activity.

One test procedure using MIESSY, for example, is the determination of the physical half-life of various radionuclides with 8 detectors simultaneously. Fig. 2.24 shows an example of Tc-99m (T1/2 = 6h) with a total measurement time of 18 hours.

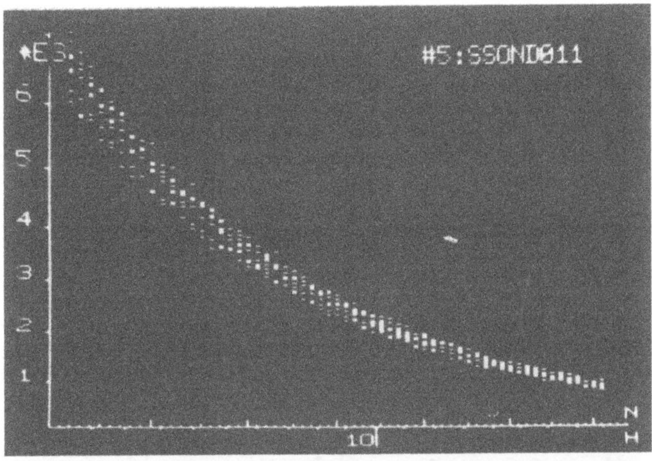

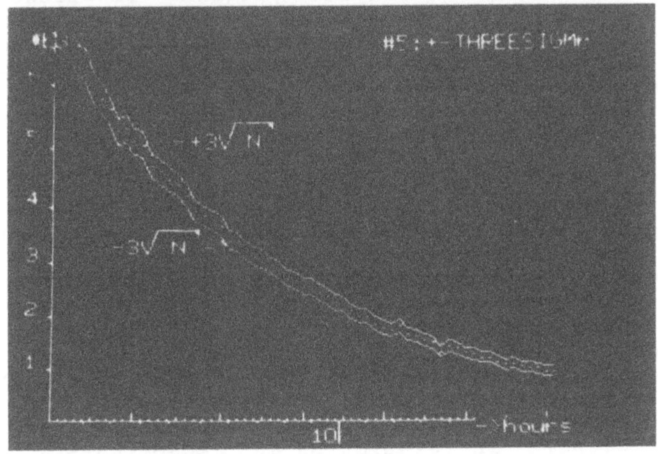

Fig. 2.24:
Top: 8 decay curves of Tc-99m after measurement with the test device for quality control
Below: one single measured decay curve (points) within ± three standard deviations (true values in that range with probability 0.997). Demonstration of the use of DISYA (see section 3.3.1.3)
Sampling interval: 18 min, counting period: 9 min, total measurement time: 18 hours

3. INFORMATION PROCESSING

The Nuclear Medical signals taken by means of suitable detectors from the nuclear radiation field emitted by the patient are abstractions of anatomical, pathological-anatomical, physiological and pathological-physiological biochemical realities. As data structures, their numerical values are reproductions of body functions with medically relevant and irrelevant constituents.

The use of digital data processing machines to solve problems in Nuclear Medicine, primarily of a numerical kind, concerns the processing of these data structures. It is the task of MIESSY to filter out the medically relevant constituents in the clinical context. Just as picture analysis is set over simple picture processing, one-dimensional signal processing requires additional analysis and interpretation for a special purpose in order to obtain medically relevant information (157).

SIMULATION and MODELING in tracer analysis of biological systems by means of mathematical models and computer programs is another aspect of problem-solving (32,33,133). Biomedical phenomena are mapped into functions and sets of algebraic differential or integral equations, the parameters of which are optimally estimated by the programs. Most compartmental models are conceived in a linear system theory context (67,96,122,183). They are great simplifications of real physiological systems and are intended to represent the relevant features of the problem under study.

COBELLI and ROMANIN-JACUR (53) present solution techniques for checking a priori structural identifiability, observability and controllability of multi-input and multi-output biological compartmental systems. This is seen as an important test of the significance of the planned input-output tracer experiment itself before radioindicators are injected and measurements taken.

Excellent program packages, such as SAAM (34) or CSMP (193), exist for the digital simulation of compartmental systems associated with the kinetics of radiotracers. General-purpose programs such as SAAM or CSMP can be very helpful in simulation and modeling studies with regard to both conceptual and computational features. Whereas huge programs of this kind are very flexible and can be applied with many options to a large variety of problems, they have to be implemented on large digital computers in centres with restrictions to the availability of interactive versions.

Information processing serves 'the solution of problems in fields of application' (117,165). Thus non-algorithmic activities (117) take their place beside programming as the link between data structures and algorithms (211). These non-algorithmic activities concern view and description of the problem as the starting point for the mutual structuring of data and algorithms, as well as the thinking up and testing of new algorithms and data structures with or without the use of ones that are already available (117). Engymetric data structures are at present mainly limited to simple numerical fields, which are associated with the measurement values of one nuclear radiation detector. With increasing clinical experience, however, more complex data structures are to be expected if the measurement values of multiple, miniaturised detectors which are attached to the body are to be analysed simultaneously ('whole body counter'). The specific a priori knowledge of the clinical physician for solving medical problems should be used via the non-algorithmic aspect of information processing (92,117,145).

If, like HARTMANN (86), one regards the process of the doctor's decision-making, recognition and judgement as a kind of search, then it is precisely information processing in dialog with the computer which permits the support of the conjectural aspect of the doctor's judgement.

Support by a computer is made easier in this non-algorithmic area of problem-solving through the dialog ability of the calculator (92,117,145,166). In addition to programming, this contains a new quality in information processing in that it permits 'reflexivity in the dialog' and 'the dialog state as the totality of stored information' (117,144,146,147).

DISYA, a dialog system for the analysis of engymetric time-activity-histograms (see section 3.3), was conceived from these ideas and from experience with the implementation of a command language for nuclear medical signal and picture processing (147,159).

Fig. 3.1 illustrates the dialog language as the highest level in the hierarchy of programming languages, being an interface between man and machine (157,159).

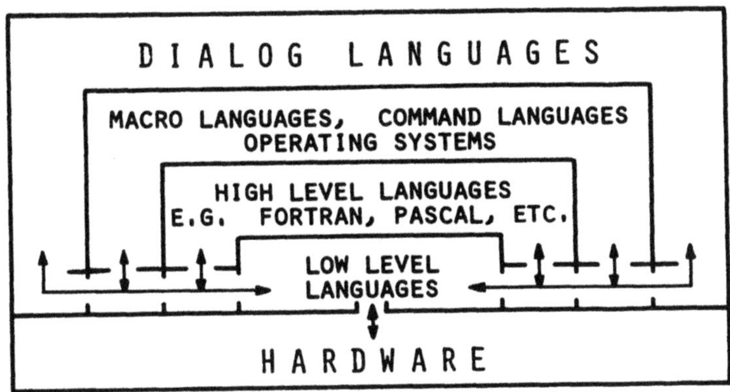

Fig. 3.1:
Language hierarchy for conversational computing

A personal-computer system (APPLE II Plus) was selected as the vehicle for DISYA in the sense of 'alternative' data processing.

3.1 'Alternative' Data Processing

The effects of electronic data processing on medicine as well as the content and significance of Medical Informatics have been investigated in detail by REICHERTZ (164,165,166,166a,166b). Immediate and comprehending use and control of computer systems by doctors in their everyday work, however, is relatively rare.

In clinical practice the question posed by PRETSCHNER (152) in 1977: 'FORTRAN - a must for doctors of Nuclear Medicine?' seems to have been given the answer 'no'. As far as is known without an exact survey, only very few of the European colleagues specialising in this subject have dealt with a higher programming language, even though the relevant courses in connection with the annual International European Nuclear-Medical Congress have been well attended (79).

Parallel to this apparent lack of acceptance, a new development which started in the USA has been under way since 1975: PERSONAL COMPUTING. It is associated with the large successes in the integration of digital microcircuit networks into micro-processors, in the development of micro-computer systems, as well as in the marketing of inexpensive 'Personal Computers'. These micro-computer systems, which are also called home, hobby, office, private, workplace, table, and compact computers, stand at the beginning of a completely new way of looking at electronic data processing, in which SCHUCHMANN (179) distinguishes four directions with programmatic goals: the psychological-pedagogic, the political-ideological, the market-political and the technical-scientific programmatic goal.

In the last of these goals the technical-scientific expert, often a layman as far as data processing is concerned, stands in the foreground. He is to be given a potent tool for his special problems. He can employ it as he likes and at any time. In contrast with the traditional centralized use and availability of comprehensive computer services in batch or time-sharing operation, there is no dependence on computer centres and personally restrictive organizational forms. Inexpensive home computers with well thought out operating systems and several higher programming languages, of which PASCAL has been particularly successful, are receiving more and more interest as semi-professional microcomputers or even minicomputers from electronic data processing experts and from industry (179,212).

Wide-ranging changes are in progress, as, for example, the 32 bit microcomputer iAPX 432 by INTEL. It must be especially noted here, and GEYER (80) draws attention to it, that the hardware concept of iAPX 432 can, as far as its structure is concerned, be transferred to the structure of the modern higher programming language ADA, although the two concepts were realised completely independently of each other (206).

The development of a DIalog SYstem for the Analysis (DISYA) of engymetric time-activity-histograms on a personal computer system in the price range < $4000 took place after experience with a dialog language as man-machine interface for algorithmic and non-algorithmic problem-solving with the mini-computers PDP 11/34, 11/55 (144,146,147,159).

3.2 Personal Computer System (APPLE II Plus)

3.2.1 HARDWARE

The system (Fig. 2.21) consists of an APPLE II Plus Personal Computer with 48k RAM, the APPLE Language System which increases the addressed memory (RAM) to 64 kbytes, a Floppy Disk II subsystem with two drives (2 Megabit/diskette), a black and white TV monitor, a colour video monitor, a printer, and a parallel interface card for the primary storage module. The system is based on the 6502 microprocessor with 56 instructions and an address field of 2^{16} at a frequency of 1.023 MHz, a 16 bit parallel address bus and a bidirectional 8 bit parallel data bus (16). A quartz was exchanged, and slight modifications were made to the hardware for colour video operation with any colour TV set available on the market (CCIR STANDARD, PAL). This is not necessary when using the euroversion. The black and white monitor is preferred to the colour graphics with 6 programmable colours when routine work is being done.

3.2.2 SOFTWARE

The software for the analysis of engymetric time-activity-histograms in dialog (DISYA), which is described separately in Section 3.3, is embedded in the diskette-oriented operating system APPLE-PASCAL. It relies to a large extent on UCSD-PASCAL by BOWLES (45). The development of DISYA was completed with version 1.1 of the operating system (3,4,12,14,15). The programming languages used are PASCAL, FORTRAN 77, and 6502 ASSEMBLER (4,12,13,15). In addition, the library of special service programs is employed. This includes the colour graphics with 53289 matrix elements (x = 279, y = 191).

APPLE-FORTRAN 77 (13) which is used is a standard subset of ANSI-FORTRAN 77 (11,102). It contains considerable improvements on the old ANSI-FORTRAN IV - 1966 (10). In addition, APPLE-FORTRAN 77 offers extensions to the official standard language. The general I/O with direct, sequential, unformatted or formatted access is performed with OPEN and CLOSE. In the computed GOTO, it is possible to use expressions for the output of a WRITE statement and in the specification for the unit I/O number. Type conversion from INTEGER to CHARACTER and vice versa is possible. COMPLEX and DOUBLE PRECISION are not defined as a restriction to the 6 data types permitted in FORTRAN 77. Further details are to be found in the APPLE-FORTRAN Language Reference Manual (13).

There are also slight differences between APPLE-PASCAL (4,15,125) and Standard PASCAL (97). As far as possible, only the standard language was employed during software development. This means that portability of most of the programs is guaranteed. Portability is not given for the use of special APPLE extensions, especially in the case of the graphics package, TURTLEGRAPHICS. Examples of its use in text and graphics are Figs. 3.11 - 3.14, which are photographed, like many others, from the screen. Special importance was attached to modularity (58,62,65,66,85,113). Development took place according to the principles of structured programming, which is supported in particular by the language structure of PASCAL (63,98,114,125,195,213).

3.3 DIALOG SYSTEM FOR ANALYSIS OF ENGYMETRIC TIME-ACTIVITY-HISTOGRAMS (DISYA)

The goals for the development of DISYA arose from practical experience in clinical and scientific Nuclear Medicine. The aim was to define a tool for physicians of Nuclear Medicine and scientists with the following specifications:

1. interactive non-algorithmic problem-solving in dialog as a new quality in information processing
2. interactive access to as large a library of algorithmic problem-solving modules as possible
3. free programmability in the higher programming languages FORTRAN and PASCAL for use in dialog
4. autonomy with independence, as far as equipment and personnel are

concerned, from the usual diagnostic equipment of Nuclear Medicine, as well as from computer centres, departmental computers and other computers widely used in Nuclear Medicine on the basis of the new engymetric system, all at reasonable cost

5. stress on the individual doctor-patient relationship with the least possible interference by the anonymous apparatus of big modern clinics and huge centres.

3.3.1 STRUCTURE AND MODULAR CONCEPT

Fig. 3.2 shows schematically the embedding of a DISYA command processor within the surroundings of the selected computer system.

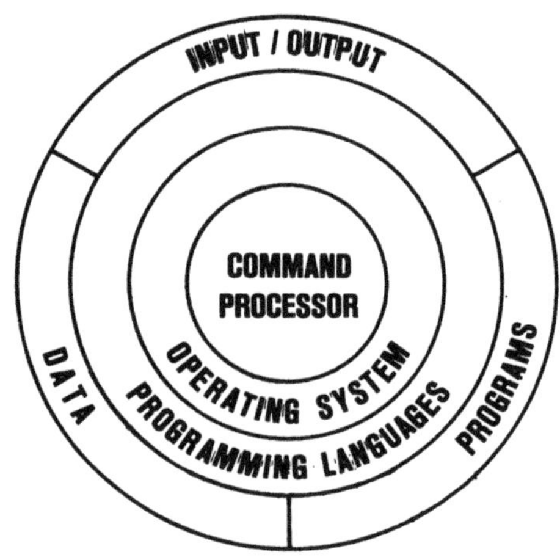

Fig. 3.2:
Scheme of the environment of the command processor of the dialog system

The standard operating system of APPLE II Plus on the basis of UCSD-PASCAL (3,14,45) serves as the operating system.

The main program of DISYA is coded in PASCAL while applying techniques of structured programming (44,45,62,66,85,98,195,210). FORTRAN is employed for special modules, e.g. spline interpolation, differentiation, Fourier transformation and the gamma variate fit (47,102). The reading-in routine for taking over data from the primary storage unit is written in ASSEMBLER.

While Fig. 3.2 shows the general environment of DISYA, Fig. 3.3 explains its special modular structure.

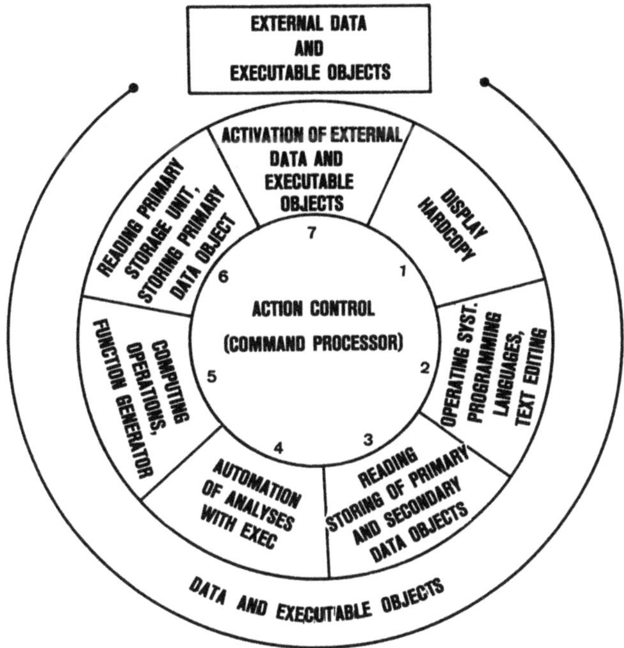

Fig. 3.3:
Modular structure of the DIalog SYstem for Analysing (DISYA) engymetric time-activity-histograms. The amount of data and executable objects (computational resources (206)) can be extended interactively, and is symbolised by the open ring at the top.

According to Fig. 3.3 there are 7 main routes of action control for problem-solving in dialog. They permit access to 58 interactions (Figs. 3.4-3.6, consecutive numbering in the box, top right). The 7 main actions are:

1. Immediate display of the desired curves (1 - 10) on the screen and/or output on the printer with the possibility of freely inserting alphanumerics into the curve display.
2. New programs can be written. Text editing and general data organisation actions can be completed via the command level of the general operating system. The change to the command level of the DISYA dialog is effected by calling up dialog.
3. Reading and secondary storing on diskette of the primary data dealt with in a dialog session with the possibilitiy of adding alphanumeric commentary. In additon, data from various primary files can be mixed.
4. Through the preparation of EXEC files, protocols that have been clinically successful can run automatically.
5. Application of monadic and dyadic computing operations to the curves. Special functions can be generated by a function generator for test purposes.

6. Reading out of the primary memory unit and taking over the original measurement values take place separately with special safety mechanisms. The original data in the primary file can only be read, but not written by DISYA.
7. External objects, which are at first not defined for the current session, can be activated in the dialog through interactive extension of the menu without extra compilation or linking the whole program.

The entire action control of MIESSY is included in the 3 command trees of Figs. 3.4-3.6. Individually, the 58 interactions schematised in these figures are explained in sections 3.3.1.1 - 3.3.1.8

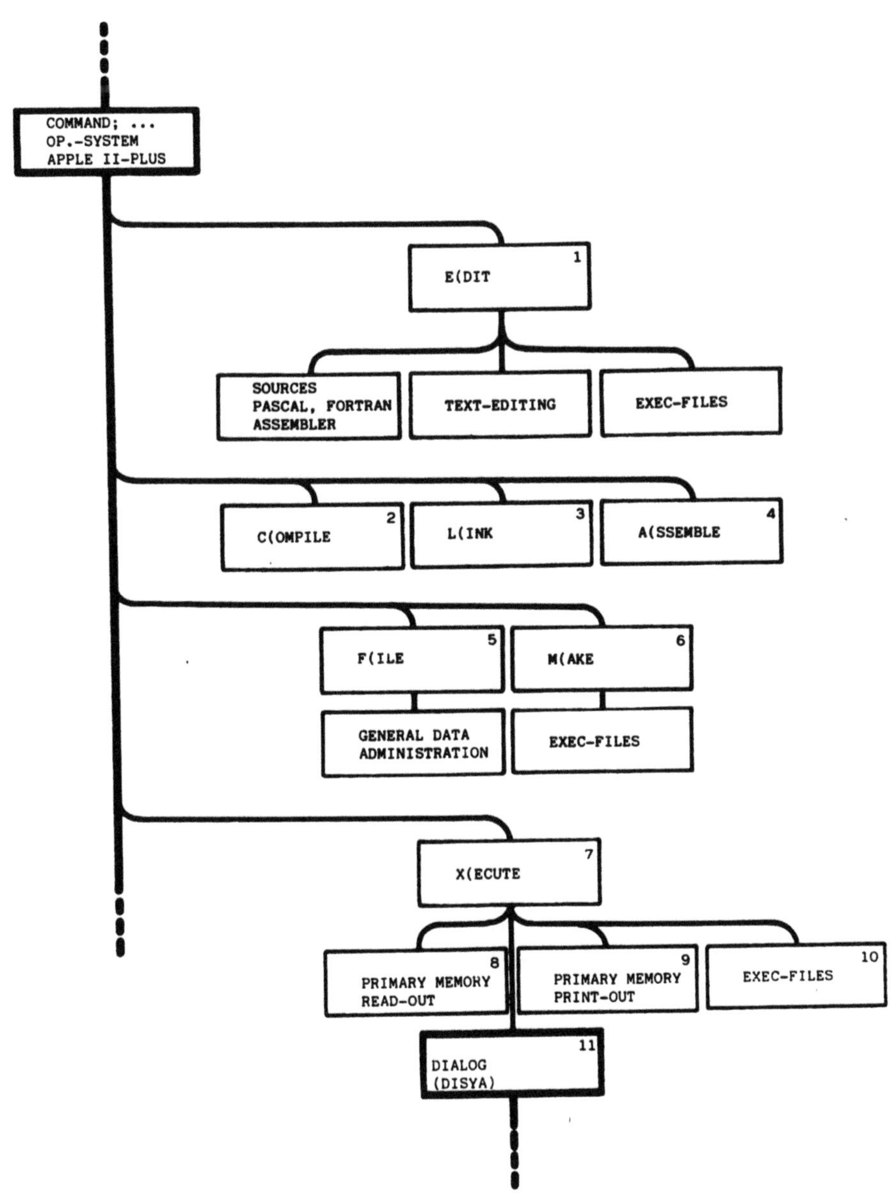

Fig. 3.4:
Excerpt from the command tree of the APPLE II Plus operating system with the most important actions with regard to MIESSY

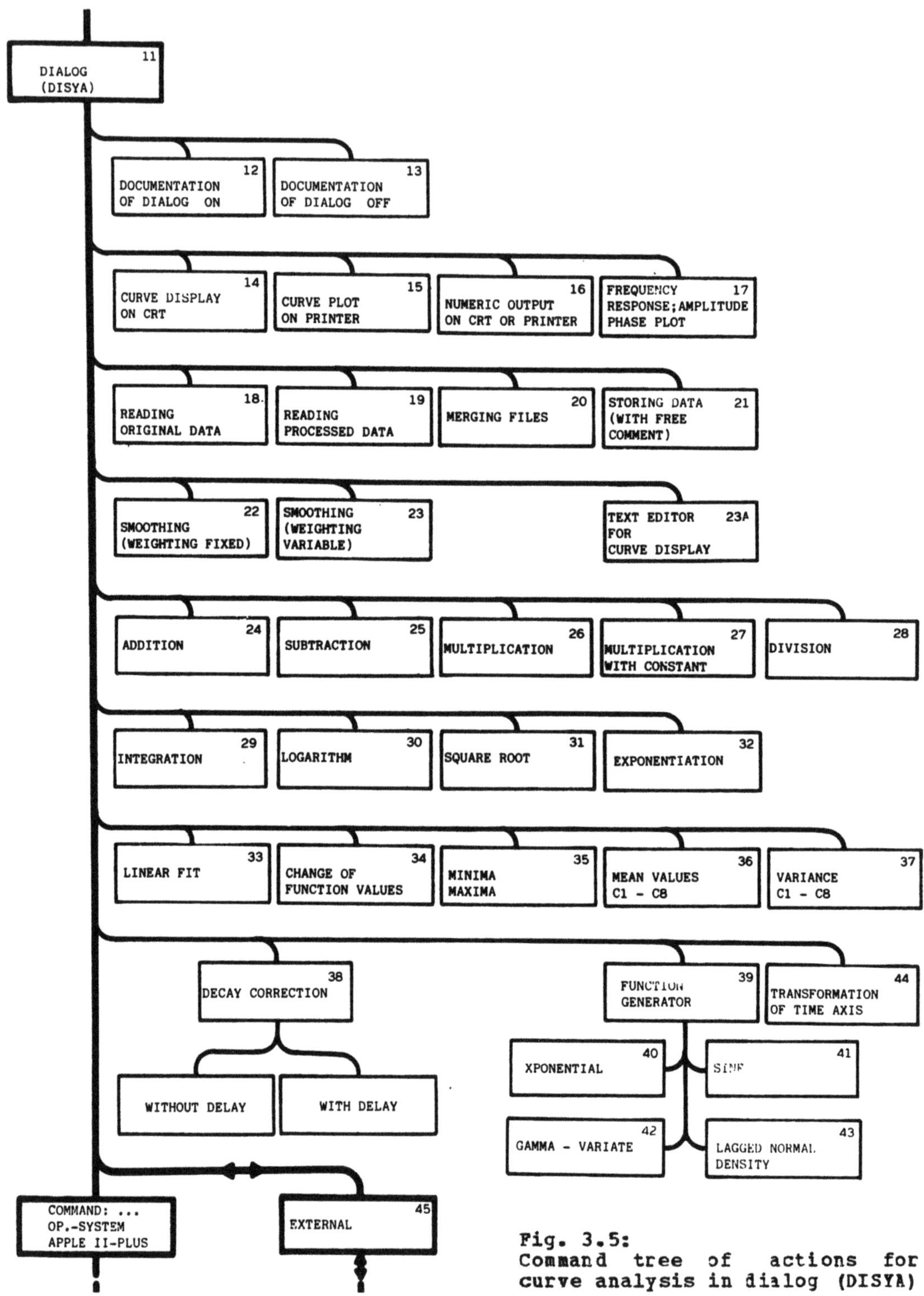

Fig. 3.5: Command tree of actions for curve analysis in dialog (DISYA)

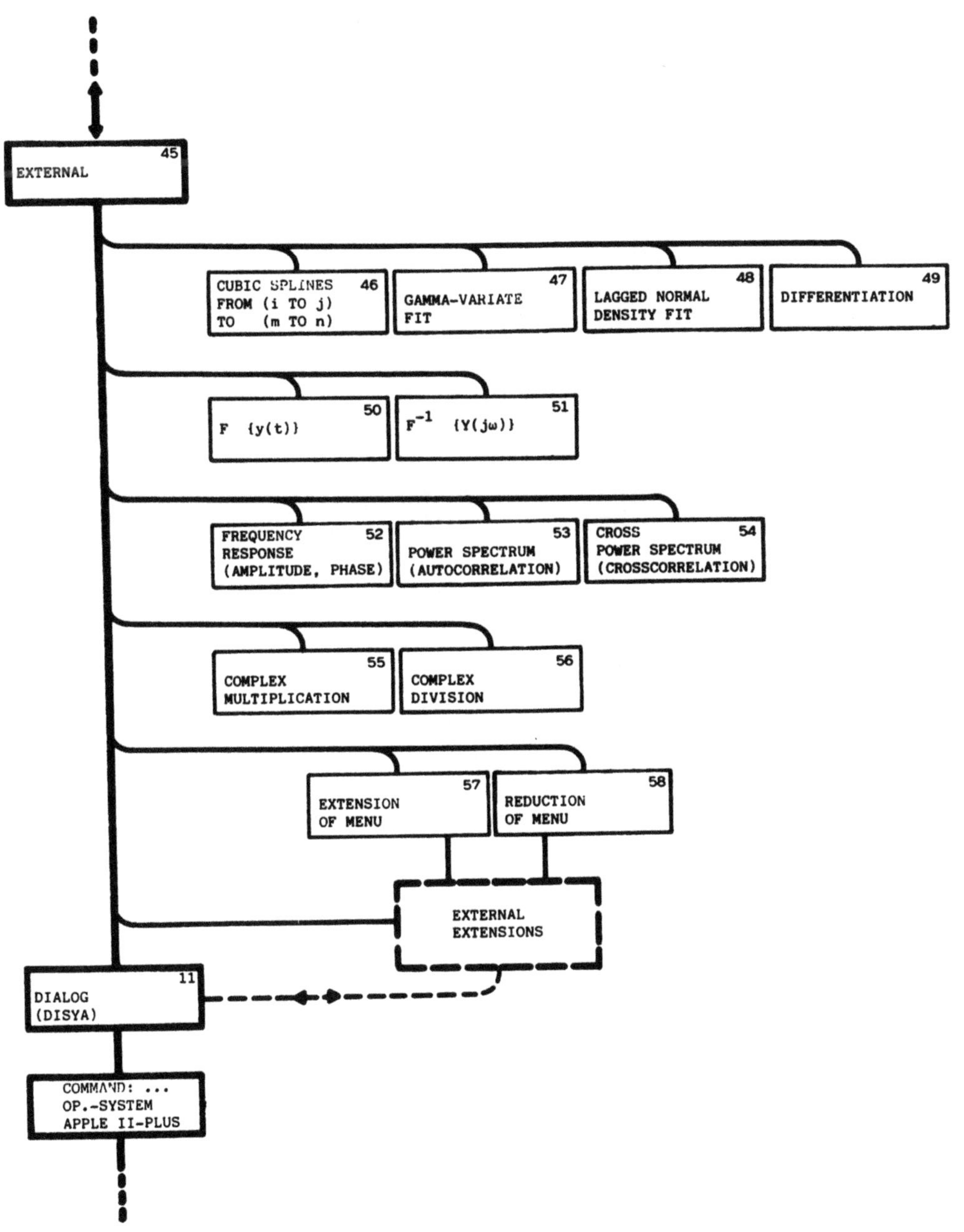

Fig. 3.6:
Command tree for curve analysis in dialog (DISYA). External extensions

The menu of Fig. 3.7 is at the basis of interactive actions. It contains commands that are available with mnemonic abbreviations.It appears on the screen before command input by the user. The abbreviations therefore do not have to be specially learnt. A new menu is generated for external extensions (see section 3.3.1.8).

```
COMMANDS:

  G(ET      R(EAD     ME(RGE    SA(VE
  DI(SP     SP(EC
  A(DD      S(UB      M(ULT     CM(ULT  D(IV
  EX(TR     CH(ANGE   Z(KOR
  MI(TT     V(AR
  L(N       E(XPO     SQ(RT     I(NTEG
  PR(INT    PL(OT     PLE(RQ
  DOC       NDOC      TIM       CHAIN
  SM(TH     GL(ATT
  F(UNK     LI(N
  Q(UIT    [T(EXT ONLY DURING DI(SP]
```

Fig. 3.7:
Basic menu with commands. Input of characters in front of the opening bracket starts an action

The rough structure of the main program DIALOG represented for the user by the commands of the menu on the screen (Fig. 3.7) is shown in the Nassi-Shneidermann-Diagram of Fig. 3.8.

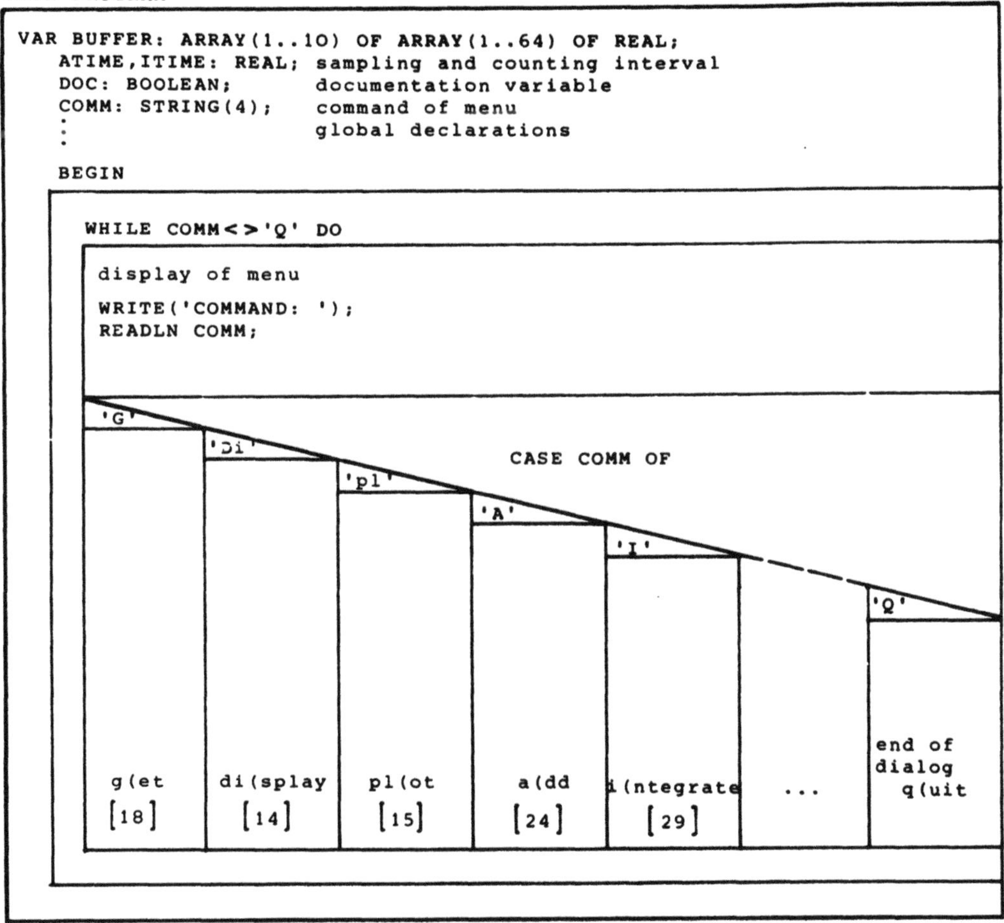

Fig. 3.8:
Structure of the main program

3.3.1.1 Command level of the general operating system (APPLE II Plus)

Fig. 3.4 shows the main actions for MIESSY, which are started from the command level of APPLE's operating system. In the following (sections 3.3.1.1 to 3.3.3) the numerals in the square brackets behind the description of the command refer to the numerals in the top right-hand corner of the boxes in the command trees (Figs. 3.4-3.6). They do not refer to the literature cited with rounded brackets.

The letters in front of the rounded opening bracket are accepted by the command processor as abbreviations. This notation, which is similar to UCSD-PASCAL (45,125), is used for uniformity. The operating system commands concern general data administration (F(ILE [5]), programming, compiling and linking in the programming languages ASSEMBLER, PASCAL, FORTRAN (A(SSEMBLE[4], C(OMPILE[2]), L(INK[3]) and the production and editing (E(DIT[1]) of source programs. Detailed descriptions are to be found in the manuals (3,4,12,14,15).

X(ECUTE [7] activates the executable objects:

```
primary memory read-out (E1      [ 8]),
primary data print out  (PR      [ 9]),
EXEC files              (...     [10]), and the
DISYA dialog            (DIALOG  [11]) (Fig. 3.7).
```

3.3.1.2 Reading, writing, mixing of data

The primary data object consists of

- the original measurement values of the 4 channels from the portable primary storage unit
- two values of time (sampling and counting interval)
- data about the patient examined:
  positioning of radiation detectors on or in the patient's body
  type of nuclear radiation detector
  dosage, type and form of application of the radioindicator
  general information about the patient
- free text

This information is asked for by program E1[8] according to a fixed schedule. It is typed interactively from the console (Fig. 2.22). The naming of the primary data object as a diskette file (3 blocks with 512 bytes) and its administration in data banks is carried out according to the rules of the operating system. As a protective measure it can only be read by DISYA, but not modified. The declaration of this object as a typical PASCAL type is shown in Fig. 3.9. Fig. 3.10 shows the corresponding PASCAL syntax diagram (97).

```
          VAR PATIENT: FILE OF RECORD
                   ID:  RECORD
                              NAME: STRING(20);
                              DATE: STRING(10);
                              SMPLINT: CHAR;
                              CNTGPRD: CHAR;
                              ST: REAL;
                              CD: REAL;
                              TIM1: STRING(3);
                              TIM2: STRING(3);
                              NUCLIDE: STRING;
                              COMMENT: STRING;
                        END;
              CHANNEL:  RECORD
                        C1,C2,C3,C4: ARRAY(1..64)OF INTEGER;
                        END;
          END;
```

Fig. 3.9:
Declaration of primary data object as structured type in PASCAL, corresponding to PASCAL syntax diagram of Fig. 3.10

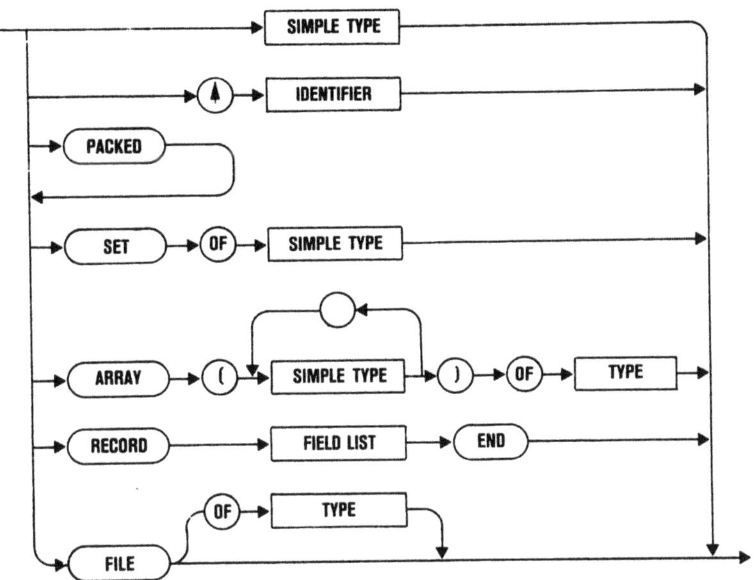

Fig. 3.10:
PASCAL syntax diagram for declaration of data types

Details of the sophisticated concept of data type in PASCAL can be found in the original 'Pascal User Manual and Report' by JENSEN and WIRTH (97). For differences from this 'Standard Pascal' language introduced in UCSD PASCAL and APPLE PASCAL see refs. (12,14,15,45,125). For further applications refs. (44,45,125,210,211) are recommended.

The command for reading the primary data object is G(ET[18]. Volume and file name are asked for when this procedure is being executed. This information is typed at the console controlled on CRT. After reading from diskette, patient and acquisition data, as typed in when reading the primary storage device, are projected on to the screen for control and positive patient identification. A current data object, consisting of 4 fields (real) with original measurement values and 6 free fields (real) is generated (Fig. 3.11). Thus 10 working buffers are available as operands for the dialog session.

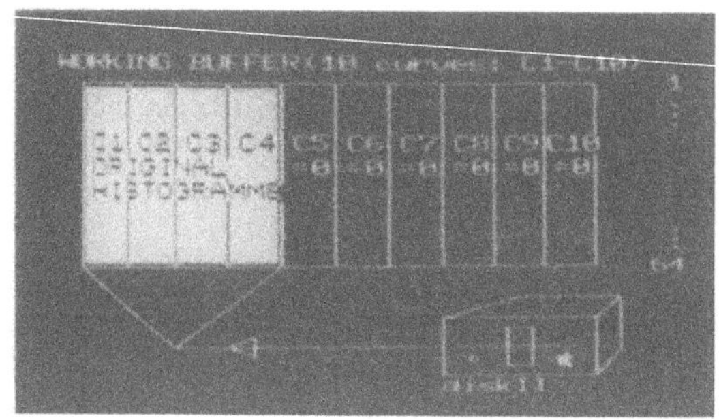

Fig. 3.11:
Reading of the original measurement values from secondary storage (diskette). They are taken from the primary data object into the first 4 arrays of the working buffer with 10 predefined arrays

The actual dialog state with regard to the curves, original and processed, and comments can be stored at the end of a dialog session on a diskette under another file name with command SA(VE[21]. This data object has a slightly different structure than the primary data object of Fig. 3.9 (activated with command G(ET[18]). The modified primary data object is of a structured type as well. It can be read again with command R(EAD[19] (Fig. 3.12).

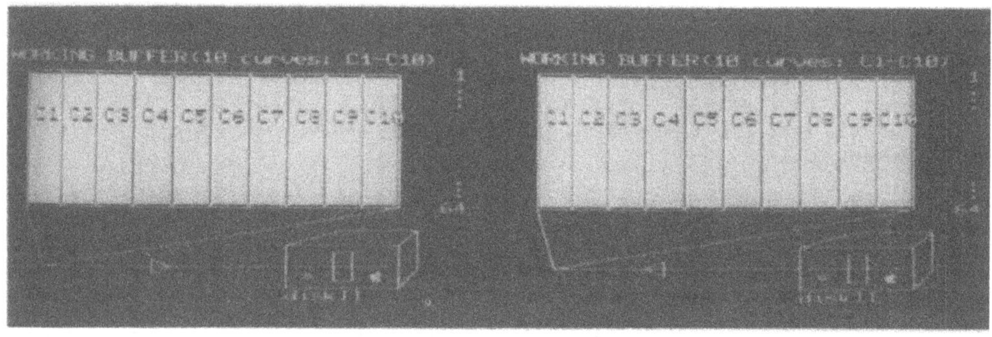

Fig. 3.12:
Storing (left) and reading (right) of processed engymetric curves, represented by two data objects of structured type

M(ERGE[20] permits the interactive mixing of engymetric curves from the same or different patients, the curves or part of the curves coming from different data objects with different file names (Fig. 3.13).

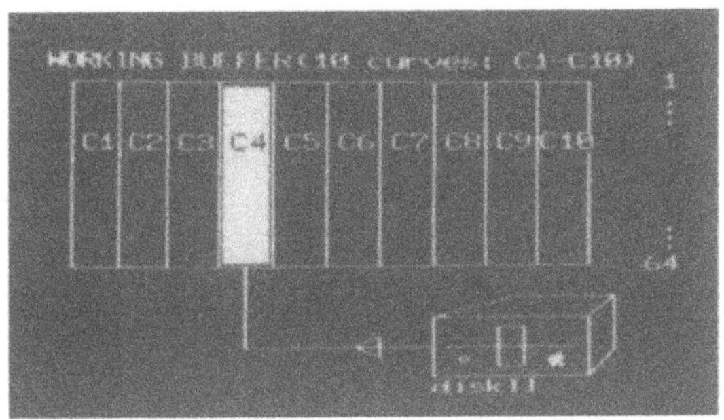

Fig. 3.13:
Mixing of data. Curve #n,n=1,...,10 from file X is read into the actual working buffer. Only one curve is read into working buffer #4

Summarized, the I/O commands are:

G(ET [18]　　M(ERGE [20]
R(EAD [19]　　SA(VE [21]

The actual dialog state is automatically stored when external extensions are called. With the return to the basic menu an automatic reading procedure takes place, making the data available again unchanged, so long as they have not been changed externally. When the DISYA level is actually left with command Q(UIT, the latest dialog state is automatically stored on diskette and read in again when DISYA is called up, after a cold start, for example.

3.3.1.3 Basic operations with time-activity-histograms

The computations realized in DISYA refer primarily to arithmetic functions, both monadic and dyadic. The time-activity-histograms can be regarded as one-dimensional vectors. The operations defined operate on these arrays in an element-by-element manner.

Logical and comparative functions as provided by APL (101), for example, have not been implemented. There has been no need for this so far during the applications.

The following are available as simple arithmetic operations on the time series C1 - C10 in the working buffer (Fig. 3.14), the numbers in the square brackets referring to the command tree in Fig. 3.5:

A(DD [24] addition of two curves
S(UB [25] subtraction of two curves
M(ULT [26] multiplication of two curves
C(MULT [27] multiplication with a constant C. With C = 0 curves, or part of them, can be deleted
D(IV [28] division of two curves
LN [30] natural logarithm $\log_e N_k$
SQ(U [31] square root
EXP [32] exponentiation
I(NTEG [29] 'integration', an adding procedure from i=m to i=n

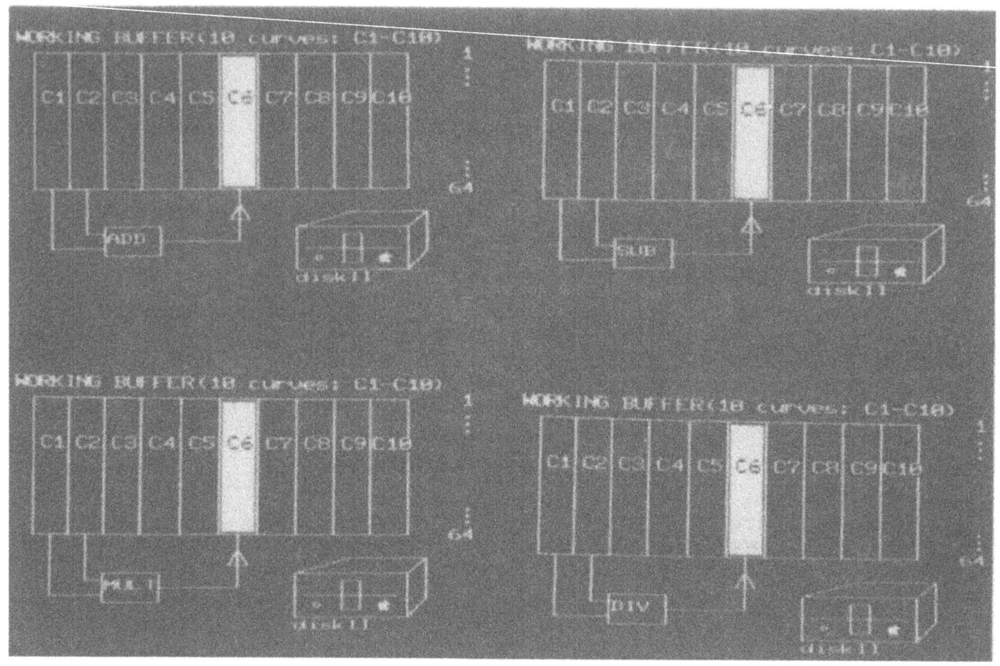

Fig. 3.14:
Illustration of curve arithmetic in DISYA. As examples, results of the respective operation on operands from the first two arrays C1, C2 in the working buffer are put into array C6

As examples of two program modules Figs. 3.15 and 3.16 show the Nassi-Shneiderman diagrams for division and the subroutine procedure used.

Fig. 2.24 demonstrates the use of the DISYA commands SQ(U[31], C(MULT[27], A(DD[24], S(UB[25], DI(SP[14], T(EXT[23A] applied to the counting statistics of one measured decay curve of Tc-99m. The 99.7 percent confidence interval is shown.

```
SEGMENT PROCEDURE DI;
VAR I, C1, C2, C3, FROM, UPTO:INTEGER;
                         SCH :INTEGER;
BEGIN
  BEGIN  (*DIALOG*)
    PAGE (OUTPUT);
    WRITELN ('C U R V E   D I V I S I O N');
    WRITELN ('----------------------------');
    WRITELN ('C3 := C1/C2');
    WRITELN;
    REPEAT
      WRITE  ('C1 ? ');
      READLN (C1);
    UNTIL  (IORESULT=0) AND (C1≥1) AND (C1≤10);
    REPEAT
      WRITE  ('C2 ? ');
      READLN (C2);
    UNTIL  (IORESULT=0) AND (C2≥1) AND (C2≤10);
    REPEAT
      WRITE  ('C3 ? ');
      READLN (C3);
    UNTIL  (IORESULT=0) AND (C3≥1) AND(C3≤10);
    REPEAT
      WRITE  ('FROM ? ');
      READLN (FROM);
    UNTIL  (IORESULT=0) AND (FROM≥1) AND (FROM≤64);
    REPEAT
      WRITE  ('UPTO ? ');
      READLN (UPTO);
    UNTIL  (IORESULT=0) AND(UPTO≥1) AND (UPTO≤64) AND (FROM≥UPTO);
  END  (*DIALOG*);
  DIV;

  (DOC=1) AND (SCH=0)
  No:
  Yes:
    BEGIN  (*COMMAND DOCUMENTATION*)
      REWRITE (EPSON,'PRINTER:');
      WRITELN (EPSON);
      WRITELN ('CURVE DIVISION');
      WRITELN (EPSON,'C',C3,'<--','C',C1,'/C',C2);
      WRITELN (EPSON, 'FROM', FROM, 'UPTO', UPTO);
      CLOSE (EPSON);
    END  (*COMMAND DOCUMENTATION*);
```

Fig. 3.15:
Nassi-Shneiderman diagram for division of curves in PASCAL. Dividing only segments of curves (from i to j) is possible

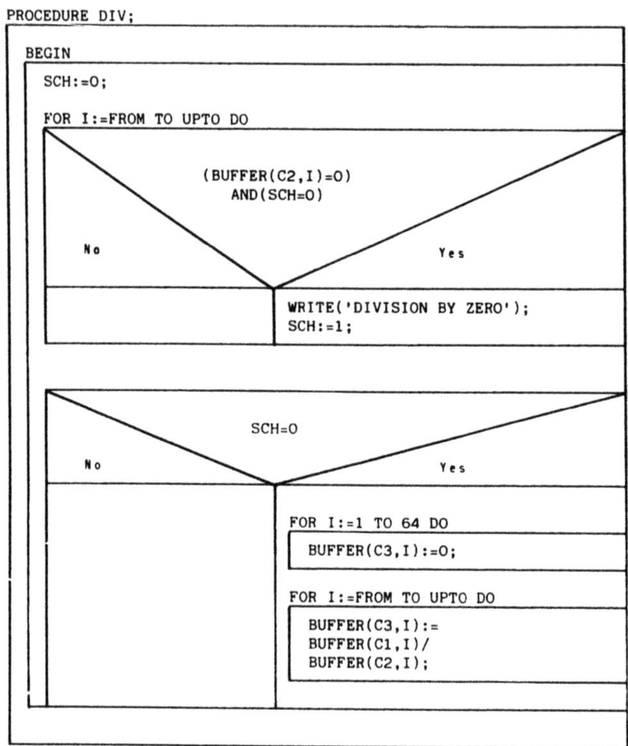

Fig. 3.16:
Diagram for subroutine procedure DIV used in the program of Fig. 3.15

All measurement values can be changed at will either individually or in groups by the command CH(ANGE [34].

Extreme value determinations (maxima, minima) with corresponding points of the time axis are given by means of E(XT [35].

Decay correction is possible with and without delay: Z(KOR [38]. For correction without delay

$$C_i = c_i \; e^{\left(\frac{(t_i \ln 2)}{t_{phys}}\right)} \tag{3.1}$$

C_i corrected countrate at time t_i, c_i measured countrate at time t_i, t_{phys} physical halflife

Decay correction with delay means correction of measurement series recorded some time t_d after injection of the radioindicator.

$$C_i = c_i \, e^{\left(\frac{(t_i+t_d)\ln 2}{t_{phys}}\right)} \qquad (3.2)$$

Before computing C_i the exponent is controlled for plausibility to see that it lies between boundary values. A clinical application of decay correction is shown in Figs. 4.4, 4.14.

Mean values M(ITT [36] and variance V(AR [37] of every function value of the first 8 time-activity-histograms C1 - C8 can be deposited in the working buffer arrays C9 and C10. The algorithm is conceived in such a way that old mean values and variances are taken into account with the addition of new curves. This means that mean values and variances can be determined at all points of registration time for practically any number of measurement series.

Smoothing, Digital Filtering.

When smoothing (moving average) time-activity-histograms c_k, k=1,...,N with error-reducing power R (105) digitally and non-recursively

$$\bar{c}_i = \sum_{k=-m}^{m} w_k \, c_{i-k} \qquad (3.3)$$

It is assumed (105) that $\bar{c}_i$ is computed only from original raw data c_i which have not been smoothed already. The number m of weighting factors w_k is odd (2m+1). In addition

$$w_{-k} = w_{+k} \qquad 0 \leq k \leq m \qquad (3.4)$$

$$\sum_{k=-m}^{m} w_k = 1 \qquad (3.5)$$

When engymetric time-activity-histograms consisting of i=64 measured countrates c_i are smoothed, the first and last data points cannot be neglected. KENDALL (105) gives a procedure for calculating weighting factors with error-reducing power and without neglecting the beginning and ending function values. A polynomial equation of degree m is fitted to 2m+1 function values. Assuming m=3, as realized in the operator SM(TH [22]

$$f(t) = a_0 + a_1 t + a_2 t^2 + a_3 t^3 \qquad (3.6)$$

is fitted to the original measurement.

Minimizing

$$\sum_{i=-3}^{3}\left(c_{t_i} - f(t_i)\right)^2 \tag{3.7}$$

leads to

$$a_o = \frac{1}{21}\left(-2c_{t_{-3}} + 3c_{t_{-2}} + 6c_{t_{-1}} + 7c_{t_o} + 6c_{t_{+1}} + 3c_{t_{+2}} - 2c_{t_{+3}}\right) \tag{3.8}$$

and the 7 symmetric weighting factors

$$(w_{-3},\ldots, w_3) = \frac{1}{21}\,(-2,\ 3,\ 6,\ 7,\ 6,\ 3,-2) \tag{3.9}$$

for the moving average.

Any number of symmetric weighting factors can be found with this procedure. The weighting factors are not symmetric for the beginning and ending values

$$t_1 \ :\ \frac{1}{42}\ (\ 1,\ -4,\ 2,\ 12,\ 19,\ 16,\ -4\ ) \tag{3.10}$$

$$t_2 \ :\ \frac{1}{42}\ (\ 4,\ -7,\ -4,\ 6,\ 16,\ 19,\ 8) \tag{3.11}$$

$$t_3 \ :\ \frac{1}{42}\ (-2,\ 4,\ 1,\ -4,\ -4,\ 8,\ 39) \tag{3.12}$$

so that the first and last 3 smoothed engymetric time-activity-histogram values become

$$\overline{c}_1 = \frac{1}{42}\,(\,39c_1 + 8c_2 - 4c_3 - 4c_4 + c_5 + 4c_6 - 2c_7) \tag{3.13}$$

$$\overline{c}_2 = \frac{1}{42}\,(\,8c_1 + 19c_2 + 16c_3 + 6c_4 - 4c_5 - 7c_6 + 4c_7) \tag{3.14}$$

$$\overline{c}_3 = \frac{1}{42}\,(\,-4c_1 + 16c_2 + 19c_3 + 12c_4 + 2c_5 - 4c_6 + c_7) \tag{3.15}$$

$$\overline{c}_{62} = \frac{1}{42}\,(\,c_{58} - 4c_{59} + 2c_{60} + 12c_{61} + 19c_{62} + 16c_{63} - 4c_{64}) \tag{3.16}$$

$$\overline{c}_{63} = \frac{1}{42}\,(\,4c_{58} - 7c_{59} - 4c_{60} - 6c_{61} + 16c_{62} + 19c_{63} + 8c_{64}) \tag{3.17}$$

$$\bar{c}_{64} = \frac{1}{42} (- 2c_{58} + 4c_{59} + c_{60} - 4c_{61} - 4c_{62} + 8c_{63} + 39c_{64}) \quad (3.18)$$

With this smoothing procedure using a third degree polynomial, the error-reducing power charging the variance of additive noise is shown in Fig. 3.17 (106).

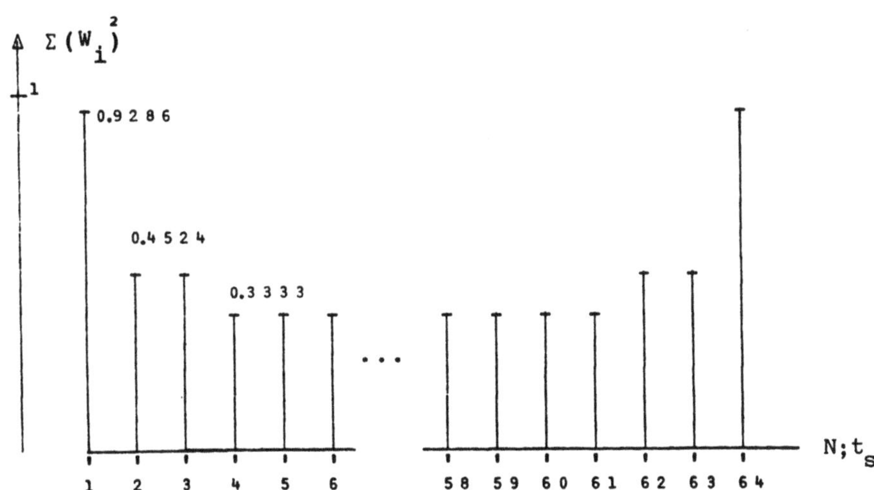

Fig. 3.17:
Error reducing power after smoothing with cubic polynomial for the 64 sampling intervals of an engymetric curve (106)

The variance is reduced by R = 0.9 at the first and last function values, and by R = 0.3 from the fourth to the sixty-first, resulting from the weighting factors of equation 3.3 (106).

The moving average smooth given above is a non-recursive digital filter and can be regarded as a linear time invariant system operator

$$\bar{c}_i = \Omega\left\{c_i\right\} = \sum_{k=-m}^{m} w_k \; c_{i-k} \quad (3.19)$$

The command SM(TH [22] initiates the above smoothing procedure using a cubic polynomial and fixed weighting factors.

With command GL(ATT [23] the weighting factors of a 3-, 5-, or 7-point smooth can be chosen interactively. The factors need not be symmetric.

The action commands in this section are summarized as follows:

A(DD	[24]	LN	[30]	CH(ANGE	[34]
S(UB	[25]	SQ(U	[31]		
M(ULT	[26]	EXP	[32]	M(ITT	[36]
C(MULT	[27]			V(AR	[37]
D(IV	[28]	E(XT	[35]		
				SM(TH	[22]
I(NTEG	[29]	Z(KOR	[38]	GL(ATT	[23]

3.3.1.4 Display, hardcopy

The command DI(SPLAY [14] permits the simultaneous, graphic representation of from one to ten 'curves'. Normalization to the maximum of a set of curves as well as scaling of the time axis according to real time during acquisition of the data take place automatically. For positive identification every curve representation contains the actual file name in the top right-hand corner. One single curve can be represented as points or with straight line elements connecting the points. White on a black background, or black on white are both possible. Photographs are taken with a Polaroid camera direct from the screen, as documented throughout this book. Free text can be inserted by calling a text editor [23A] from the DISYA menu. Hardcopy of the measurement series 1-10 is possible on the printer with PL(OT [15] or as numeric output PR(INT [16]. Representation of frequency characteristics with the abscissa in Hertz (sec^{-1}) is possible as well, both on the screen or on the printer with command PLF [17] (see Fig. 3.18).

Documentation of the dialog itself on the printer takes place after typing DOC[12]. This command is retracted with NDOC [13].

The commands of this section are:

DI(SP	[14]	DOC	[12]
PL(OT	[15]	NDOC	[13]
PR(INT	[16]		
PLF	[17]		

3.3.1.5 Function Generator

The function generator activated with the command F(unction [39] of the basic menu produces trigonometric sine [41], single exponential [40], and gamma variate [42] functions $f(t_i)$ of the forms

$$y_A(t_i) = k_1 \sin k_2 t_i \tag{3.20}$$

$$y_B(t_i) = k_3 \ e^{-k_4 t_i} \tag{3.21}$$

$$y_C(t_i) = k_5 \ (t_i - t_a)^{k_6} \cdot e^{-k_7 (t_i - t_a)} \tag{3.22}$$

Parameters k_i, $i=1,\ldots,7$ and t_a (appearance time) are asked for by the program module as well as the number of the working buffer in order to store the curve, so that from there it can be displayed and controlled on the screen.

Display of the curves is limited to i=1,...,64 sampling points. One way of overcoming limitations imposed by the number i of discrete values of the independent variable t_i is by cubic spline interpolation (see section 3.3.1.6). In addition, the range of the time axis can be transformed at will with the command TIM [44]. This module asks for a scaling factor and changes the time axis to any range, keeping it as a global variable for further computations if, for example, segments of engymetric curves have been extended or compressed using cubic splines.

Apart from the gamma variate (eq. 3.22) to describe indicator dilution curves in applications in Nuclear Medicine, the lagged normal density equation (eq. 3.25, 3.26) has been an attractive descriptive mathematical model (25,56,87). It represents one ideal mixing cell with a transport delay (87).

As BASSINGTHWAIGHTE et al. (25) show, it is the convolution of a Gaussian normal density curve

$$f(t) = \frac{1}{\sigma\sqrt{2\pi}} e^{-\frac{(t-\mu)^2}{2\sigma^2}} \tag{3.23}$$

and a single exponential

$$g(t) = \frac{1}{\tau} e^{-\frac{t}{\tau}} \tag{3.24}$$

It can be described by the convolution integral

$$h(t) = f(t) * g(t) = \int_0^t f(u)g(t-u)du \tag{3.25}$$

or equivalently by a non-homogeneous differential equation

$$h(t) = \frac{1}{\sigma\sqrt{2\pi}} e^{-\frac{(t-\mu)^2}{2\sigma^2}} - \tau \frac{dh(t)}{dt} \tag{3.26}$$

The parameters are τ for the time constant of the monoexponential (eq. 3.24) and σ for the standard deviation of the normal density curve with median μ (eq. 3.23). Quantities such as mean transit time $\bar{t} = \mu + \tau$ (the first moment), and variance $\sigma^2 + \mu^2$ (the second moment), are easily calculated from the parameters (21,25,87). The mathematical notations (3.23-3.26) assume continuous variables (t), though, like equations (3.20-3.22), for use with IISYA variables are always discrete $f_j(t_i)$. Thus to avoid misunderstandings, both notations are used as usual.

With a total measurement time of 192 sec, which allows for equidistant sampling intervals of t_s= 3 sec, Fig. 3.18 shows applications of the function generator.

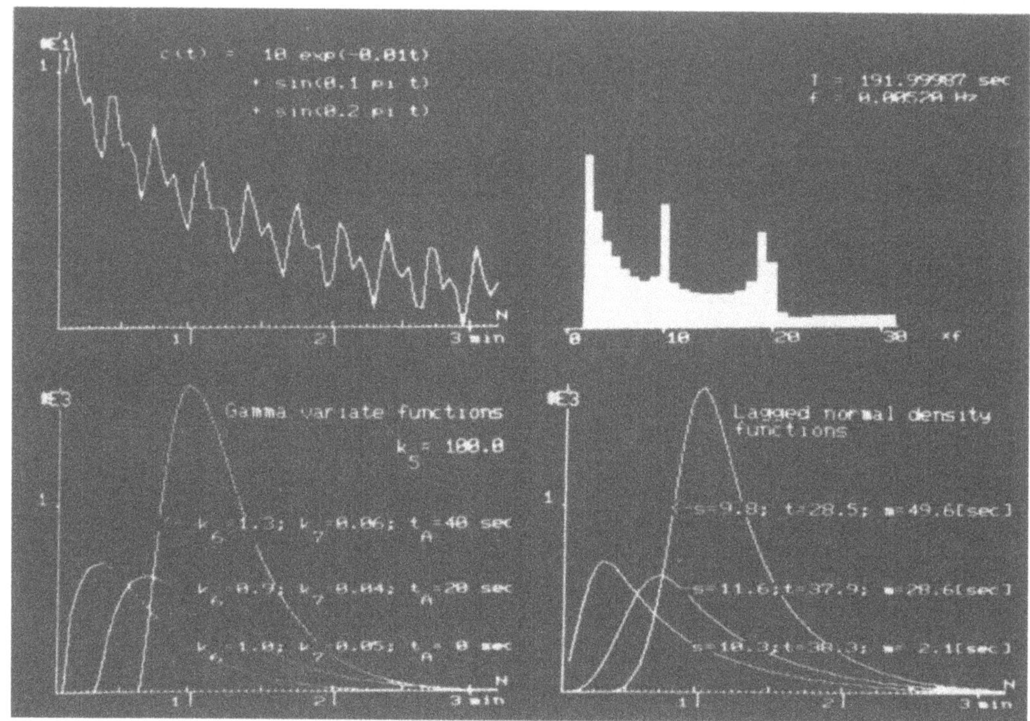

Fig. 3.18:
Examples from the function generator; amplitude spectrum
Top: sum of one exponential and two sines (left), with their amplitude spectrum
Bottom: gamma variates (left), lagged normal density functions
Parameters according to eqs. 3.20 - 3.22, 3.26. Range of time axis uniformly set to 192 sec with sampling interval t_s =3 sec
(s= σ , m= μ , t=τ)

The commands of this section are

```
F(UNC  [39]    with  E(XPO   [40]
                     S(INE   [41]
                     G(AMMA  [42]
                     L(AGGED [43]
```

3.3.1.6 Curve fitting procedures

Time-activity-histograms can be fitted in DISYA linearly, with single exponentials, gamma variate, and lagged normal density functions. Complete measurement sequences are thus condensed into a few single numbers, the estimates of appropriate parameters. The coefficient of variation v can be used as a measure of goodness of fit (25,110).

$$v = \sqrt{\frac{\sum_{i=1}^{N}(c_i - e_i)^2}{N-1} \cdot \frac{N}{\sum_{i=1}^{N} c_i}} \tag{3.27}$$

e_i being the measured discrete engymetric and c_i (t_i) the computed time sequence.

The linear fit is by the usual least squares method.

Exponentials

To fit a curve to a single exponential, its logarithm is taken by LN [30]. A least squares linear fit LIN [33] results in a straight line with slope k_4 and intercept ln k_3 (eq. 3.21).

Sums of exponentials with only a few terms, as in most applications, can be fitted by curve peeling if the decay constants differ by factors of at least two (96). The exponential term with the smallest k is approximated first by means of least squares fitting after the logarithm [30] has been taken. EX(ponentiation [32] and S(ubtraction [25] from the original measurement series is the first step in the peeling process, which is then repeated for the other terms.

Gamma-variates

To estimate the parameters of the nonlinear gamma-variate function eq. 3.22 is first linearized by taking logarithms. A weighted least squares analysis with weights inversely proportional to the error variance leads to the estimate of the parameters of the model (151).

Before regression analysis, however, the appearance time t_a has to be approximated. This is accomplished after SM(oothing [22] once and searching for the longest positive slope using cubic spline interpolation. Fig. 3.19 shows the results of fitting the lagged normal density curves of Fig. 3.18 to gamma-variates.

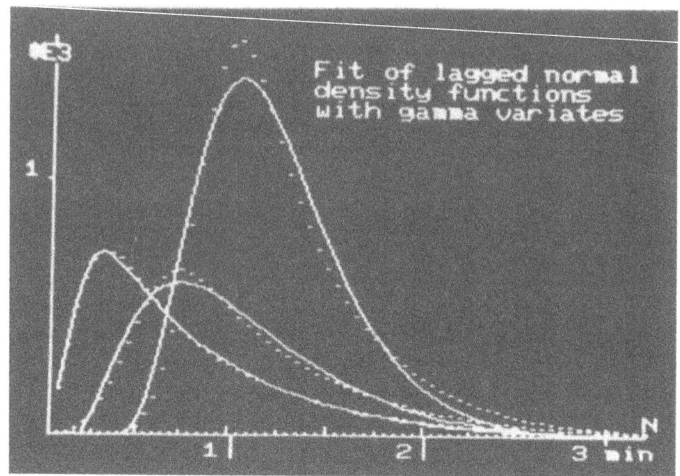

Fig. 3.19:
Three approximations of lagged normal density (points) with gamma variate functions (lines)

Lagged normal density functions

In order to optimize the computed approximation of measured time series with the lagged normal density curve (eqs. 3.25, 3.26), a method described by KNOPP and BASSINGTHWAIGHTE (110) has been programmed for interactive use.

For each iteration the coefficient of variation v (eq. 3.27) between measured curve and calculated model is taken to define a 3-D surface above the plane of two model parameters. As Fig. 3.20 shows for one curve, the extremum with the smallest coefficient of variation is taken for the best fit of a lagged normal density applied to the gamma variate functions of Fig. 3.18.

The program is called via EXTERNAL [45]. Execution time depends on the first estimates of the parameters that the search begins with. The results of fitting 3 gamma variate functions of Fig. 3.18 with lagged normal density curves are shown in Fig. 3.20. The coefficients of variation for the approximations are $v_1 = 0.14$, $v_2 = 0.16$, $v_3 = 0.16$.

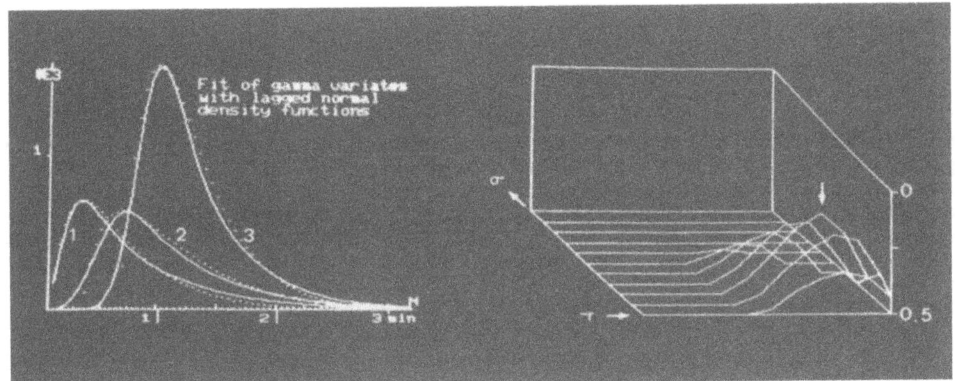

Fig. 3.20:
Approximation of gamma variates (points) of Fig. 3.18 with lagged normal density functions (lines). All parameters are given in Fig. 3.18. For curve #2 coefficients of variation are plotted on the right over σ,τ-plane with v =0.16 (arrow) for the final fit (110)

Interpolation with cubic splines

This procedure [46] matches the engymetric time series piecewise - continuously by means of cubic polynomials (167). It is used for shifting, compressing and extending engymetric curves. The extensions like interpolative 'magnifying' serve other operations, such as the differentiation [49] or finding the appearance time t_a of the gamma variate function. Compressing, extending, and shifting mean that engymetric time series from different measurements can be combined.

The problem consists of finding a cubic polynomial

$$y_i(t) = a_i + b_i(t-t_i) + c_i(t-t_i)^2 + d_i(t-t_i)^3 ; \quad i = 1,2,\ldots, N \quad t_i \leq t \leq t_{i+1} \tag{3.28}$$

for the engymetric measurement series e_i (t_i), i=1,2,...,N.

The sampling intervals t_s are equidistant $t_{i+1} - t_i$ = const. There are constraints for values and derivatives at the fixed interval ends of the independent variable t_i.

With

$$y_{i-1}(t) = a_{i-1} + b_{i-1}(t-t_{i-1}) + c_{i-1}(t-t_{i-1})^2 + d_{i-1}(t-t_{i-1})^3 \tag{3.29}$$

and conditions

$$y_{i-1}(t=t_i) = y_i(t=t_i) \tag{3.30}$$

$$\dot{y}_{i-1}(t=t_i) = \dot{y}_i(t=t_i) \tag{3.31}$$

$$\ddot{y}_{i-1}(t=t_i) = \ddot{y}_i(t=t_i) \tag{3.32}$$

$$\ddot{y}_1(t=t_1) = \ddot{y}_N(t=t_N) = \emptyset \tag{3.33}$$

the system of equations is solved for coefficients a_I , b_I , c_I , d_I .

The interactive application of the module for interpolation with cubic splines [46] via EXTERNAL [45] is demonstrated in Fig. 3.21. The program first asks for the number of the curve in the actual working buffer which is to be interpolated. Then the segment range of its independent variable (from i to j) which is chosen for interpolation is typed at the console. By default this interval is extended to the total range of 64 'sampling points', i.e. those that can be displayed with DISYA (from m=1 to n=64).

If the default correspondence between the segment of the independent variable is not chosen, the program asks for the mapping range explicitly (from m to n). Fig. 3.21 shows an example of compressing and shifting, Figs. 4.24, 4.25 show applications with extension ('magnifying') and shifting for the estimation of ventriculo-peritoneal shunt flow with drained hydrocephalus.

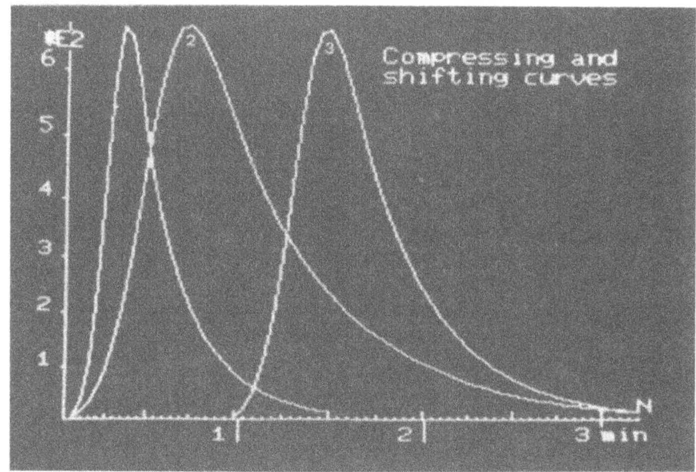

Fig. 3.21:
Compressing and shifting curve #2 of Fig. 3.20 from (i=1 to j=64) to the left (m=1 to n=30) and asymmetrically to the right (m=20 to n=64) (3) using cubic splines

With the ME(RGE [20] option it is possible to append different measurements with different counting t_c and sampling periods t_s , resulting in one curve only.

The combined single curve segments are adapted for the overall measurement time T_N with the aid of the module for transformation of the time axis [44]. This is necessary if one is looking for the approximation of one total curve consisting of different segments from different engymetric long-term measurements at the same place but at different times.

Diverse counting periods t_c are corrected by constant multiplication [27] and one must be aware of changing statistics.

The linear approximation is accessible from the basic menu LI(N [33]. The other curve fitting procedures are called via

EXTERNAL [45] with numbers (1) CUBIC SPLINES [46]
(2) GAMMA VARIATE [47]
(3) LAGGED NORMAL DENSITY [48]

3.3.1.7 External extensibility during dialog sessions

The external extensibility of the DIALOG [11] is performed via the command EXTERNAL [45] of the basic menu. Subsequently, the actual dialog state with regard to the data is stored on the diskette. A menu appears with the actions that currently can be carried out externally. First, the menu contains the commands for EXTENSION [57] and REDUCTION [58] of this menu. The extension command allows for the addition of completely new executable objects without having to leave the main program.

The operating system (version 1.1 (3,4)) provides for a UNIT CHAINSTUFF in the SYSTEM.LIBRARY file. Via this UNIT one program can chain to another program with or without passing parameters. Fig. 3.22 shows the PASCAL source statements and messages for the compiler of a small program called 'CONSTANT1P'. It sets all the function values of one curve equal to 1.0, its working buffer number being asked for interactively.

```
(*$S++*)
PROGRAM CONSTANT1P;
USES CHAINSTUFF;

TYPE SAVEAREA = ARRAY (1..10) OF ARRAY (1..64) OF REAL;
     COMMON   = RECORD

                  TIME:REAL;
                  KAN :SAVEAREA;

                END;

VAR IO:FILE OF COMMON;
    I,K:INTEGER;

BEGIN (*CONSTANT1P*)

PAGE(OUTPUT);
WRITELN('ALL FUNCTION VALUES = 1.0');
WRITELN('------------------------');
(*$I-*)
REPEAT

  WRITE('WHICH CURVE ? ';
  READLN(K);

UNTIL (K≥1) AND (K≤10) AND (IORESULT=0);
(*$I+*)

RESET(IO,'COMMON');
GET(IO);

FOR I:=1 TO 64 DO
              IO^.KAN(K,I) :=1;

PUT(IO);
CLOSE(IO,LOCK);

SETCHAIN('DIALOG');
END.
```

Fig. 3.22:
Example of an external PASCAL program called CONSTANT1P. It sets all the function values of one curve to 1.0 and chains back to the main program (SETCHAIN ('DIALOG'); last line before END.)

The program of Fig. 3.22 can be called from the DIALOG [11] via EXTERNAL [45] after EXTENSION [57] of the external menu. After having been executed it automatically passes control back to the DIALOG menu with the procedure SETCHAIN ('DIALOG').

This option of the Apple PASCAL language makes it possible to chain main programs. In Fig. 3.23 two main programs execute alternately. They have access to one diskette file COMMON for data exchange.

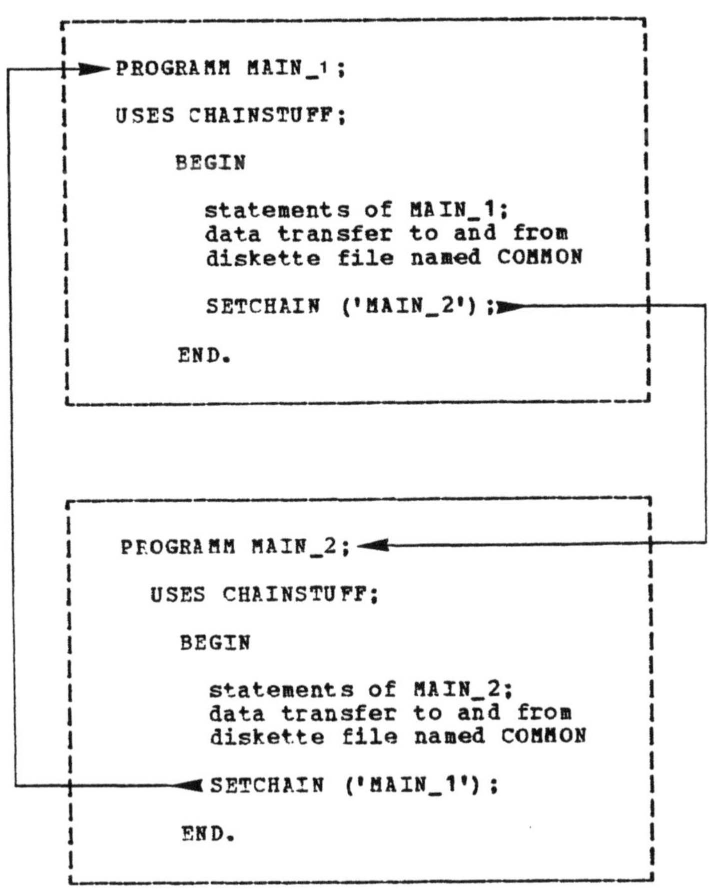

Fig. 3.23:
Chaining of two main programs with mutual data exchange using one diskette file COMMON

UNIT CHAINSTUFF permits the chaining of PASCAL programs only. If one defines a PASCAL carrier for BILINGUAL applications, FORTRAN programs can be used as well. The PASCAL carrier program is responsible for the dialog with the user and the chaining in connection with UNIT CHAINSTUFF.

The data interface for the FORTRAN program is a diskette file named COMMON in the example of Fig. 3.24. Just like the pure PASCAL source program of Fig. 3.22, the BILINGUAL example program consisting of a FORTRAN source inside its PASCAL carrier sets the values of one curve equal to 1.0 (Fig. 3.24).

```
(*$S++*)
PROGRAM CONSTANT1F;
(*$U#5:FCHAIN.CODE*)
USES UFCHAIN;
(*$U#4:SYSTEM.LIBRARY*)
RTUNIT,CHAINSTUFF;

VAR I,K: INTEGER;

BEGIN (*CONSTANT1F*)
PAGE(OUTPUT);
WRITELN('ALL FUNCTION VALUES = 1.0');
WRITELN('-------------------------');
(*$I-*)
REPEAT

  WRITE('WHICH CURVE ? ');
  READLN(K);

UNTIL (K≥1) AND (K≤10) AND (IORESULT=0);
(*$I+*)

RTINITIALIZE;
FCHAIN(K);
RTFINALIZE;

SETCHAIN('DIALOG');
END.


      SUBROUTINE FCHAIN(I)
      DIMENSION FIELD(10,64)
C
      OPEN(1,FILE='COMMON',STATUS='OLD',FORM='UNFORMATTED')
      READ(1) DT
      READ(1) ((FIELD(K,J),J=1,64),K=1,10)
      CLOSE(1,STATUS='KEEP')
C
      DO 10 K=1,64
      FIELD(I,K) = 1.
10    CONTINUE
C
      OPEN(1,FILE='COMMON',STATUS='OLD',FORM='UNFORMATTED')
      WRITE(1) DT
      WRITE(1) ((FIELD(K,J),J=1,64),I=1,10)
      CLOSE(1,STATUS='OLD')
C
      RETURN
      END
```

Fig. 3.24:
Example of a bilingual external program consisting of a PASCAL carrier and a FORTRAN program

In this way programs have been developed for operations such as discrete Fourier transformation (DFT) [50], the inverse (IDFT) [51], complex multiplication [55] and division [56], power spectrum [53], cross power spectrum [54], curve interpolation using cubic splines [46], first derivative via splines [49], curve approximation with gamma variate [47] or lagged normal density function [48] (see command tree of Fig. 3.6).

A new data object is provided for the complex calculations in connection with Fourier transforms. Fig. 3.25 shows the correspondence of time and complex frequency domain as well as the operations defined with complex numbers.

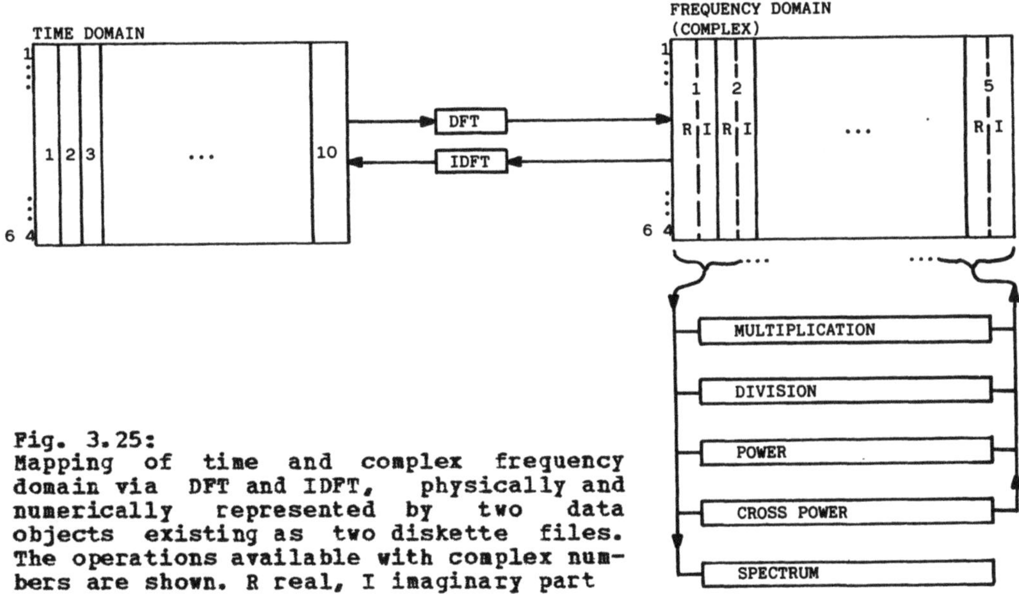

Fig. 3.25:
Mapping of time and complex frequency domain via DFT and IDFT, physically and numerically represented by two data objects existing as two diskette files. The operations available with complex numbers are shown. R real, I imaginary part

The implemented actions arrived at with EXTERNAL [45] are summarized in Fig. 3.6.

3.3.1.8 Exec-files

To a large extent, the actions of DISYA already described correspond with those of a command language (159,196). All the additional possibilities of a dialog language in an extended sense, which according to KUPKA and WILSING, PFEIFFER, PRETSCHNER and PFEIFFER (117,144,147,159) contain, for example, control structures and expressions, are not explicitly defined in DISYA. If necessary, their implementation occurs implicitly in the objects that can be executed (85).

A succession of instruction sequences using the commands of the command tree of Figs. 3.4-3.6 can be 'frozen' after they have proved clinically successful as one single 'program'. This executable object is called an EXEC-file, prepared according to the rules of the operating system (3). When being executed, the actions of each command are performed one after another in exactly the same sequence as was typed when the EXEC text file was made [6].

3.3.2 LINGUISTIC REPRESENTATION OF DISYA

An approach based on KUPKA and WILSING (117) is chosen for the formal description of the dialog system DISYA developed for the analysis of engymetric time-activity-histograms. All the present input and output grammars of all possible user inputs and system replies can be described formally and independently of each other. A summary of them leads to the definition of the global grammar G of DISYA

$$G = (V, A, P, T) \tag{3.34}$$

where

$$T: T = \{\text{initial sign}\} \tag{3.35}$$

$$A: A = \{\text{alphanumeric signs}\} \cup R_S \tag{3.36}$$

A is the set of terminal signs, and R_S is the set of the terminal, nonalphanumeric signs (e.g. time-activity-histograms as engymetric curves), with which the system reacts e.g. as computed results, error messages etc.

$$V: V = \{T, K\} \cup R_B \cup \tilde{R}_S \tag{3.37}$$

The set V is the non-terminal alphabet of G. T is the initial sign and K the set of the objects that can be executed at the present time (menu), represented by the mnemonic commands which refer to file-handling, monadic and dyadic functions etc. (see Figs. 3.4 - 3.6).

R_B is the set of all the replies given by the user as a reaction to the system inquiries with regard to the actual elements of the data object (operand). Incorrect replies also form part of this set.

$\tilde{R}_S$ is the system reaction to input from the user. The set consists of questions by the system for operands $r \in R_B$. V can be extended through the activation of new objects that can be executed externally. It can be reduced by the removal of executable objects. From the equation (3.37), however, the changeability of K through the interactive addition or erasure of external modules is not explicitly visible. The change of K in the dialog is occasioned by the calling up of an element $k_{extern} \in K$. k makes the actual menu K available for changes.

In order to add a new element a rule from P is activated, which with the subsequent input of a so far unknown command $k' \notin K$ does not lead to an error message, but to the extension

$$K := K \cup \{k'\} \tag{3.38}$$

In order for an element to be erased, a rule is activated from P, which removes the element $k'' \in K$ and which leads to a reduction of the set

$$K := K \setminus \{k''\} \tag{3.39}$$

In additon to ASSEMBLER, the higher programming languages PASCAL and FORTRAN with their own syntax structures and the operating system functions associated with them are available for the realisation of k' (13,14,15,97,102).

With this capability of flexible alteration of the set of the objects K that can be executed in the dialog without interruption of the current dialog session, there is the possibility of implementing not yet realized, but potentially interesting, routines. In addition, depending on the field of application, there is also the possibility of switching the external, currently interesting functions to the basic menu. It saves time if the interesting actions can be transferred from the external sphere to the menu K. V is defined at the time of dialog.

$$P: P = \{u \rightarrow v / u \in V,\ v \in (V \cup A)^*\} \qquad (3.40)$$

P is the production set which determines the transfers of state in the dialog. $(V \cup A)^*$ is the set of all the words over the alphabet $(V \cup A)$.

In modern languages, as for example in ADA, the traditional language constructs PROCEDURE and FUNCTON are extended by the modules ('logically related collection of resources'):

PACKAGE ('subprograms and data resources') and

TASK ('resources for concurrent programming') (206).

Thus ADA already seems to contain the conceptual possibilities of external extensions as explicit elements individual to the language, as, for example, in the module PACKAGE (206). Although these features are very convenient for the user and programmer, especially regarding modularity, they still follow the traditional concept of programming languages, and in essence they do not realize the concept of 'external extensions' aimed at with the true dialog language (147).

The EXEC function belonging to the operating system is employed to connect a number of commands to one object that can be executed under a new name (macro) for the automation of complex analyses and for batch processing (3) (section 3.3.1.8).

Whereas the vague idea of a so-called 'extensible language' might have been present in the author's mind, DISYA does not even approach the possibility of extensions by further syntactic constructs introduced by the user during a dialog session (211). Nevertheless, the concept of external objects, which may be of the (structured) data or program type, facilitates the integration of programs developed 'somewhere else', however complicated they may be, into the current biosignal processing system based on an inexpensive personal computer (159,162). The power of this form of CONVERSATIONAL COMPUTING allows one in a systematic and consistent manner to integrate analysis methods as module building blocks into a general carrier system frame. These modules can then be used interactively in clinical routine not only by computer experts but also by personnel who are not computer-oriented (147,159,162).

3.3.3 EXAMPLES OF THE USE OF DISYA

The application examples which follow are by no means original or new. They are taken from selected published data. What is new here is the ease with which models, computations, and solutions arrived at with far greater means in the original papers can be simulated and judged interactively in dialog sessions with the personal computer system. A quick and stimulating 'feeling' can be obtained for possible problem solutions arising from sophisticated, primarily non-medical, fields, but probably of some use for the medical specialist's own application. A personal computer with a dialog system and graphics seems suitable for transferring this knowledge. If one completes exercises in a dialog fashion, the results of which are seen immediately for control, this greatly helps one to study, learn, and judge new methods. NUMERICAL CONTROL of equations and their derivations has proved especially useful in detecting errors during the early stages of work, particularly in research.

The interactive aspect, the possibility of easily extending the program library in dialog, and low cost are important features in the choice of a personal computer system as the electronic data processing machinery for one-dimensional signals in Nuclear Medicine. Its interactive use can be complementary and supplementary to the passive study of papers and books.

Indicator dilution

In the study of radionuclide tracer kinetics, notions, terms, and a priori knowledge from linear system theory are widely used (19,20,21,23,26,28,49,96,122,183,220). Fig. 3.26 shows a very simple hydrodynamic input-output model system (single inlet, singe outlet) with (engymetric) detectors serving as a basis for some fundamental definitions in tracer dilution methodology (22,24,26,27,122,220). The flow F of a fluid is analysed, solutes of which are labeled for convective flux. Nonconvective fluxes produced by mechanisms other than the flow of the carrier fluid, such as diffusion, uptake by organs etc. are not taken into account.

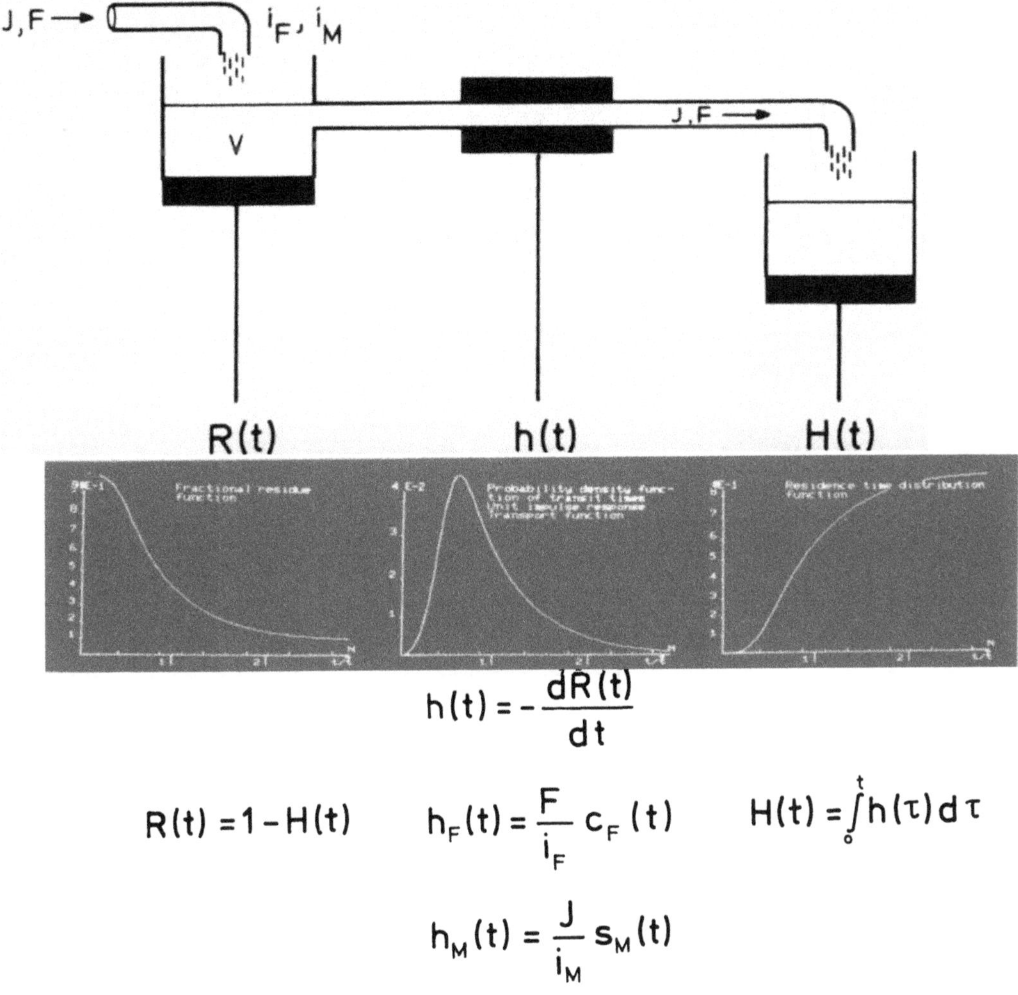

Fig. 3.26:
Idealized model system (linear, stationary) with engymetric detector arrangement and signals related to radioindicator dilution. Labeling either by constant infusion or bolus injection techniques. h(t) is assumed to be the lagged normal density curve #2 of Fig. 3.20 with unit area and mean transit time $\bar{t}$ =66.5 sec

In addition to the equations of Fig. 3.26, equations for the conservation of mass are used to derive noninvasive techniques to determine FLOWS, FLUXES, and VOLUMES of distribution by the external detection of radiation emitted by the radioindicator used (22,23,24,28,122,220).

For example, after inlet slug injection of a dose of indicator i_F labeling carrier fluid with constant flow F, the amount injected will have left the system with the time-varying concentration $c_F(t)$

$$i_F = F\int_0^\infty c_F(t)\,dt \tag{3.41}$$

For convective flux J, the mother substance M is labeled with indicator i_M and c_F (t) is substituted by the specific activity s_M (t)

$$i_M = J\int_0^\infty s_M(t)\,dt \tag{3.42}$$

Thus for flow F and flux J (122):

$$F = \frac{i_F}{\int_0^\infty c_F(t)\,dt} = \frac{h(t)_F \cdot i_F}{c_F(t)} \tag{3.43}$$

$$J = \frac{i_M}{\int_0^\infty s_M(t)\,dt} = \frac{h(t)_M \cdot i_M}{s_M(t)} \tag{3.44}$$

The equations hold for mass, volumes of distribution, and concentration. A linear correspondence, or at least a known relation, between these quantities and the engymetric signals (COUNTS/t), as described in eq. 2.1 by the integral for 3-dimensional space, has to be assumed in order to obtain some degree of isomorphism with the real world (18).

Substance Extraction

In another demonstration of the use of DISYA, sodium extraction by isolated blood-perfused dog hearts is estimated.

Methods, formulas, and original data are taken from the work of GULLER et al. (83). The indicator dilution method consists of the registration of photons from a non-permeating reference tracer (I-131 albumin) and from a diffusible radioindicator (Na-24 Cl). Both are injected as a bolus into the aortic root. The emitted radiation is detected from the venous outflow and from over the intact heart, discriminating both energies. This leads to the normalized transport h(t) and residue function R(t), one pair each for the intravascular and the permeant tracer. In their paper GULLER et al. (83) show the validity of taking residue functions from the external radiation monitoring of an intact organ to estimate extraction and capillary permeability. As this seems to be an approach of general interest, their calculations are repeated with DISYA interactively (Fig. 3.27).

Extraction across the myocardial capillary bed is estimated from the venous outflow curves, the probability density functions of transit times h(t), and the residue functions R(t) obtained from monitoring the intact left ventricular wall.

Six measurement figures for extraction E(t) are taken, three from the unit impulse responses h(t), and three from the residue functions R(t). Subscripts p,n refer to time-activity-histograms from the permeating (Na-24 Cl) and non-permeating indicator (I-131 albumin).

1. integral extraction

$$E_{h1}(t) = \int_o^t [h_n(\tau) - h_p(\tau)]d\tau \tag{3.45}$$

$$E_{R1}(t) = R_p(t) - R_n(t) \tag{3.46}$$

2. instantaneous extraction

$$E_{h2}(t) = 1 - \frac{h_p(t)}{h_n(t)} \tag{3.47}$$

$$E_{R2}(t) = 1 - \frac{\dot{R}_p(t)}{\dot{R}_n(t)} \tag{3.48}$$

3. area-weighted extraction

$$E_{h3}(t) = \frac{\int_o^t [h_n(\tau) - h_p(\tau)]d\tau}{\int_o^t h_n(\tau)d\tau} \tag{3.49}$$

$$E_{R3}(t) = \frac{R_p(t) - R_n(t)}{1 - R_n(t)} \tag{3.50}$$

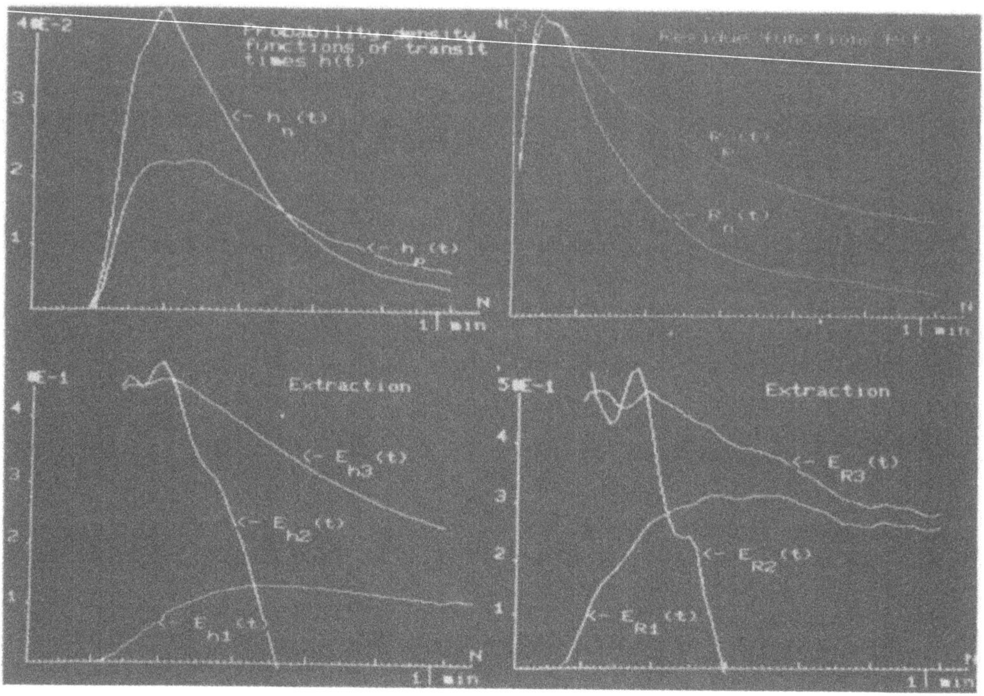

Fig. 3.27:
Top row: original measurements taken from GULLER et al. (83).
Below: calculated extractions according to eqs. 3.45-3.50

In Fig. 3.27, the top row shows the original curves $h_{n,p}(t)$ and $R_{n,p}(t)$ taken from table 1 (83,p.365) and, underneath, the calculated extraction curves. To obtain results such as these with DISYA the interactive steps are

1. typing the original measurement values into the working buffers 1-4 (Fig. 3.11)

2. performing the operations of differentiation, integration, subtraction, division with the operands in buffers 1-4 using working buffers 5-10 for intermediate results

3. display of the curves with text editing [23] for the final Polaroid photographs of Fig. 3.27

Exponentials

In parent-daughter radionuclide transformations the time course of the daughter product coming into existence through the decay of the parent radionuclide and decaying itself at the same time is described by a BATEMAN equation (169,188). It is the solution of two differential equations for mass balance. The mathematical modeling of this precursor-product system is identical to the description of one-way flow for two compartments P,D in series. The time course of specific activity at the outflow is

$$s_D(t) = \frac{m_o}{M_P - M_D}\left(e^{-k_1 t} - e^{-k_2 t}\right) \tag{3.51}$$

The injected dose of indicator into P at t=0 is m_o . The flux/mass ratios for the compartments P D are (122)

$$k_1 = \frac{J}{M_P} \quad \text{and} \quad k_2 = \frac{J}{M_D}$$

The time courses for activities s_D (t) (eq. 3.51) and

$$s_P(t) = \frac{m_o}{M_P} e^{-k_1 t} \tag{3.52}$$

are shown in Fig. 3.28.

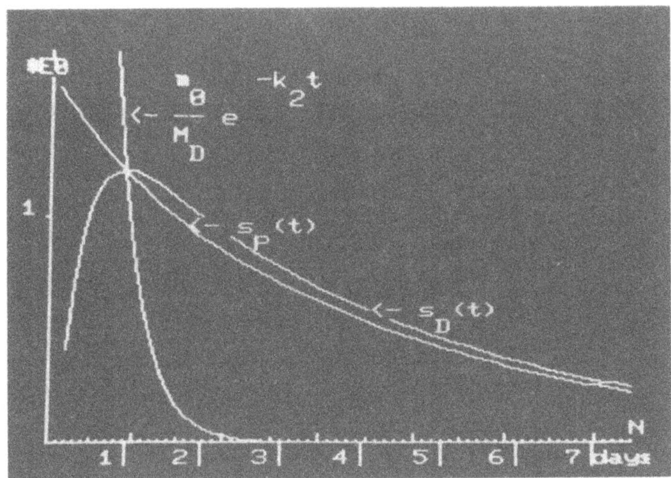

Fig. 3.28:
Computed time courses of activities in precursor-product or in two-compartment system P,D

The parameters K_1 , K_2 have been taken with a hypothetical Mo-99 (T1/2=66h) -> Tc-99m (T1/2=6h) generator in mind. The fact that only the fraction of 0.924 of Mo-99 decays for Tc-99m has been neglected (169). s_D (t) (eq. 3.51) can also be obtained by convolution of the two truncated exponentials

$$\frac{m_o}{M_P} e^{-k_1 t} * \frac{m_o}{M_D} e^{-k_2 t} = \frac{m_o\left(e^{-k_2 t} - e^{-k_1 t}\right)}{M_D - M_P} \tag{3.53}$$

The sequence of commands, with mapping into frequency domain, for DISYA (Fig. 3.25) is

1. discrete Fourier transformation (DFT) [50] of the exponentials
2. complex multiplication
3. inverse discrete Fourier transformation (IDFT) [51]

The crosscorrelation of two functions in time domain corresponds to the cross spectral density in frequency domain (46,52). Using the theorems of PARSEVAL and WIENER-KHINTCHINE

$$\Phi_{12}(\tau) = \int_{-\infty}^{\infty} e_1(t)e_2^*(t-\tau)dt \circ\!\!-\!\!\bullet\; E_1(\omega)\cdot E_2(\omega) = \Phi_{12}(\omega) \qquad (3.54)$$

the crosscorrelation sequenes of engymetric time-activity-histograms are computed.

Inverse discrete Fourier transformation (IDFT) of the cross spectral density results in the crosscorrelation function with a maximum not affected by amplitude fluctuations of the original time series. ROSEN and SILVERMAN (170) used this technique for videodensitometric measurements of blood flow. The location of the maximum of φ_{12} provides the maximum likelihood estimate of mean transit time $\bar{t}=\bar{t}_2-\bar{t}_1$ of a bolus passing two detectors.

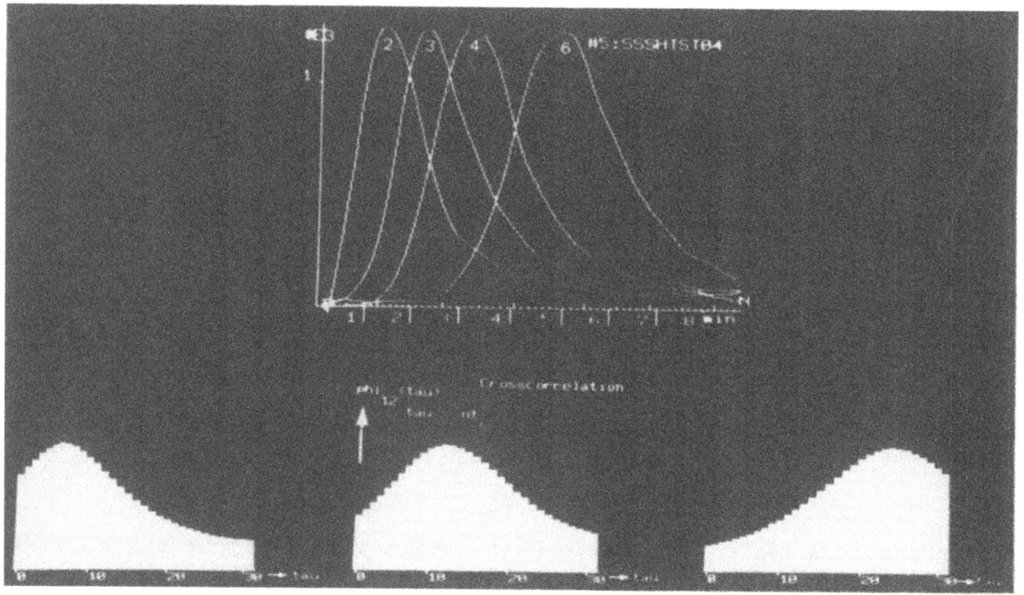

Fig. 3.29:
Crosscorrelation sequences of time-activity-histograms (top). Below from left to right: crosscorrelation of curves 2 and 3, 2 and 4, 2 and 6

The example of Fig. 3.29 is taken from the shunt-flow measurements (Fig. 4.23).

Curves 2 and 3, 2 and 4, 2 and 6 are crosscorrelated. After DFT [50] the cross power spectra are calculated [54] and transformed back into time domain [51] (Fig. 3.29). The occurrence of the maxima of the crosscorrelation sequences is multiplied by the sampling interval t_s. This leads to the difference of the mean transit times of the bolus passages under the respective detectors.

The accuracy for shunt-flow determination with this method in comparison to the procedure used in section 4.6.1 has not been tested as yet.

Mathematical operations frequently employed in the above context are Fourier transformation, convolution, deconvolution, autocorrelation, crosscorrelation etc.

Operations such as these provide a unifying mathematical approach to many different applications. The basic idea is to transform curves from their function domain into a transform domain (time to frequency) and vice versa via the Fourier transformation (1,46,52).

The Fourier transform [50] of the lagged normal density function (Figs. 3.20, 3.21) is divided [56] by the transform of the corresponding monoexponential in frequency domain. The inverse transformation [51] of the ratio leads to the normal density curve in time domain as shown in Fig. 3.30. This result corresponds to deconvolution. In terms of linear system theory it is the system transfer function that is calculated from input and output signals.

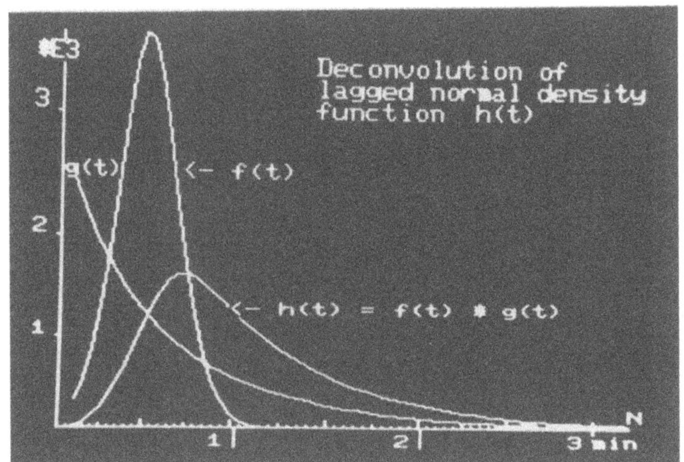

Fig. 3.30:
Deconvolution resulting from calculations in frequency domain. Normalized to the same integral

Interesting properties regarding the two domains are, for example, (46,52,122)

- convolution in time domain corresponds to multiplication in frequency domain
- the area under a function is equal to the value of its transform at origin

- the area under convolved functions is the product of areas under the factors
- abscissae of centres of gravity ('mean transit times') can be added
- variances add under convolution
- the autocorrelation function of a signal is the Fourier transform of its power spectrum

The command trees of Figs. 3.5 - 3.6 show a way of performing operations such as the above NUMERICALLY in dialog with DISYA using external extensions. The theory of one-dimensional SIGNAL ANALYSIS, the more general subject, is discussed thoroughly by BRACEWELL (46), CHEN (52), PAPOULIS (140). There are excellent books by JACQUEZ (96), SHIPLEY and CLARK (183), LASSEN and PERL (122) on tracer kinetics dealing in depth with the topics of compartmental, non-compartmental, stochastic and black box analysis.

When complex analyses such as the above are being performed, the computational power of the 8 bit machine does not always permit very short response times during dialog. It can also restrict the precision of extensive calculations. This may concern, in particular, the discrete Fourier transformations (46,52). No detailed analysis of computational errors and limits for all the algorithms used has been carried out.

The aim of the definition of MIESSY and DISYA was to create an inexpensive self-contained TOOL for the Nuclear Medicine physician, enabling him to perform medical examinations using biological data.

4. CLINICAL APPLICATIONS

It is not yet possible to perceive all the occasions when engymetry could be applied in Nuclear Medicine. The system described here, which is one that can be carried by the patient, is particularly suitable for long-term examinations. It is, however, also used just as successfully for short-term measurements, e.g. with short-lived radionuclides such as the positron emitter O-15 (T1/2 = 2 min).

Table 4.1 summarizes a number of areas in which engymetry can be of advantage in Nuclear Medicine.

1. Thrombosis (X)
2. Chronic venous insufficiency (X)
   - postthrombotic syndrome (X)
3. Compartment syndrome (X)
4. Radiocardiography (X)
   - right-to-left shunts (X)
   - left-to-right shunts (X)
5. Renography (X)
   - glomerular filtration rate (X)
   - transplant function (X)
6. Regional blood flow (X)
   - skin
   - brain (X)
   - muscle (X)
   - intraoperative (X)
   - bone (X)
   - heart
   - teeth
   - amputation level selection
7. Tumor detection
   - intraoperative detector directed dissection of tumors
8. Oviduct patency control
9. Lymph kinetics (X)
10. Hematology (X)
    - ferrokinetics
    - labeled blood cells (X)
11. Blood distribution changes (X)
12. Cerebrospinal fluid dynamics (X)
    - shunt flow (X)
13. Peripheral arterial disease (X)
14. Biorhythms of the kinetics of labeled pharmaceuticals (X)
15. Substance extraction by organs (X)
16. Absorption, long-term kinetics of labeled pharmaceuticals (e.g. I-125-NPH-insulin)
17. Regional lung ventilation, perfusion (X)
    - edema

Table 4.1:
Clinical areas in which Nuclear Medical engymetry can be employed (own experience marked by (X))

In Table 4.1 own results relating to groups of patients and casuistic examples are marked by (X). The fields of application not marked by (X) seem to be promising for engymetric measurements, or are taken from the literature on the subject. Individual applications of subsystems after Fig. 2.1 do exist, but without the conceptual unity of engymetry in the sense of MIESSY as developed here. When summarized in survey form, the fields of application from the literature are concerned with:

- KIDNEY FUNCTION DIAGNOSIS: the determination of glomerular filtration rates (41,42,148,171) and the MONITORING OF TRANSPLANTS (186,187),
- in the determination of REGIONAL BLOOD FLOW: skin (17), teeth (199), brain (123), and canine myocardium (100),
- INTRAOPERATIVE LOCATION OF TUMOR TISSUES: with Au-198 colloid the detection of macroscopically inconspicuous lymph nodes with micrometastases in nonseminomatous germinal testis tumors (8),
- RADIOACTIVE PHOSPHORUS UPTAKE TEST: 'the most reliable method for the diagnosis of malignant eye tumor' and 'the safest method for the intraoperative determination of tumor tissue in brain and spinal cord' (199),
- detection of Xe-133 in the abdomen in the control of OVARY DUCT PATENCY (143),
- early detection of BONE ABSCESSES in cases of infected tooth apices with Tc-99m-polyphosphate (76),
- determination of the ABSORPTION OF RADIOACTIVELY LABELED PHARMACEUTICALS: the subcutaneous absorption of I-125-NPH insulin (112),
- selection of lower-extremity AMPUTATION LEVEL (128)

With regard to the radioactive phosphorus uptake test to detect and localize malignant tumour tissue it is expected that dramatic progress will be made in tumor RADIOIMMUNODETECTION with antibodies. Interest is focussed especially on monoclonal antibodies. For the evaluation of their uptake and kinetics in diagnosis, and potentially in therapy, engymetric data from long-term measurements in loco, in situ might prove useful.

The radionuclides used in our own clinical applications are either on the market or are produced in the reactor or cyclotron of the 'Department of Nuclear Medicine and Special Biophysics' of the Medizinische Hochschule Hannover.

The positron emitter O-15 (T1/2 = 2 min) is produced in the cyclotron (SCANDITRONIX, max. proton energy: 36MeV) by means of N-14 (d,n) O-15 reaction with a deuteron energy of 8.5 MeV.

The bromide (Br-82) is obtained from the reactor (TRIGA Mark I) by neutron irradiation of NH_4 . For the elimination of the undesired Br-radionuclides which are additionally produced during this process, the irradiated sample is permitted to decay for 48 hours before further use.

4.1 Thrombosis Detection

Deep vein thrombosis, mostly arising in veins of the lower extremities, can be detected early by means of the radioactive fibrinogen uptake test (FUT) (104). The uptake of radioactively labeled fibrinogen into a forming or growing thrombus is detected with this typical Nuclear Medical test. After experience with the I-125 fibrinogen uptake test for the early diagnosis of leg vein thrombosis on 323 patients with alloplastic replacement of hip joints (197,208), two questions arose:

1. whether the successful FUT can also be employed for the detection of thrombosis in other blood vessels than just the leg veins, and

2. whether the assumption that most thromboses already occur during surgery (115,197,207,208) can be proved using procedures of Nuclear Medicine.

Through the development of MIESSY and small nuclear radiation detectors attached to the skin it was possible to go into these questions. With regard to the first question, the early diagnosis of the forming of thrombi in implanted vein grafts in the heart was attempted after aorto-coronary venous bypass surgery on 26 patients.

In coronary heart disease, aortocoronary venous bypass surgery is, for many selected cases, the preferred therapy for the improvement of symptoms and for increasing efficieny as well as life expectancy (126). One serious postoperative complication that is feared is the early occlusion of an implanted blood vessel through thrombosis. Developing thrombi, however, can be detected at an early stage with FUT through the intravascular deposit of radioactively labeled fibrinogen (103,104,136,149,197,208).

With regard to the second question, continuous intra- and postoperative engymetric measurements were carried out on 23 patients with neurosurgical operations of the spine. The results achieved here are discussed in Section 4.5 (intraoperative blood distribution changes).

Material and Method

After intravenous injection of 120 µci I-131 fibrinogen the precordial and temporal nuclear radiation fields were detected and counted with the portable scaler - timer of Fig. 2.5. Countrates were taken each day for 9 days following surgery at 5 measurement points on each of 26 patients who had been operated on (149). Fig. 4.1 shows diagrammatically the position of the 4 precordial measurement points. The radiation field measured temporally on the skull served as reference.

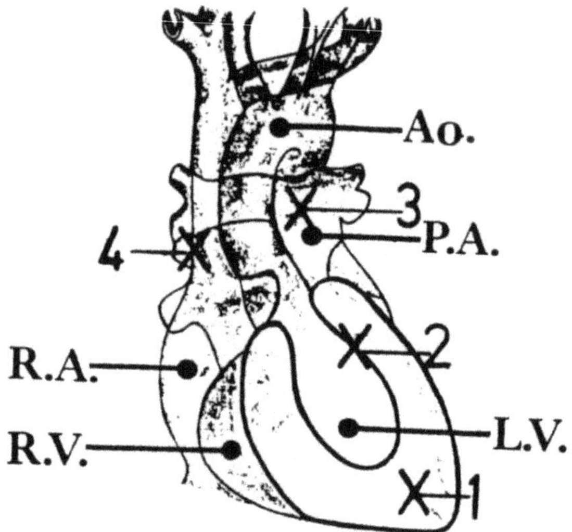

Fig. 4.1:
Location of the four precordial measurement points (1-4) for GM counter. (Ao: aorta, R.A.: right auricle, R.V.: right ventricle, L.V.: left ventricle, P.A.: pulmonary artery)

Results and discussion

Fig. 4.2 shows the time course of the ratios from the sum of the precordial and reference countrates. Two patients have an increase (+,.), which it was possible to verify coronarographically as a closure of a bypass graft.

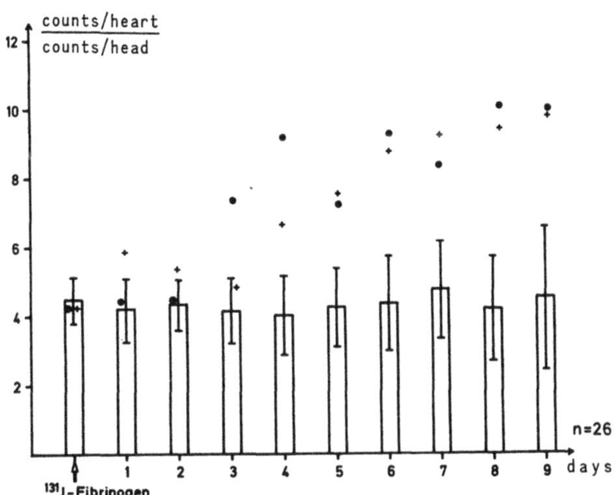

Fig. 4.2:
Results of FUT with group of patients (n=26) after aorto coronary venous bypass surgery. The increase in the ratios of 2 patients (+,.) indicates the coronarographically verified early thrombosis of a bypass graft

As an introductory example for the demonstration of pharmacokinetics with engymetry, Fig. 4.3 shows the mean course ($\pm$ 1σ) of the measured countrates representing radioactivity in volumes of head and heart regions during the period of 9 days after injection of I-131 fibrinogen. The measurement values come from the 26 postoperative patients (without the 2 cases with increasing ratios) after Fig. 4.2. Two components with a half-life period of 21 hours and a slow one of 96 hours were obtained by means of biexponential curve-peeling according to a two-compartmental model for the in-vivo kinetics.

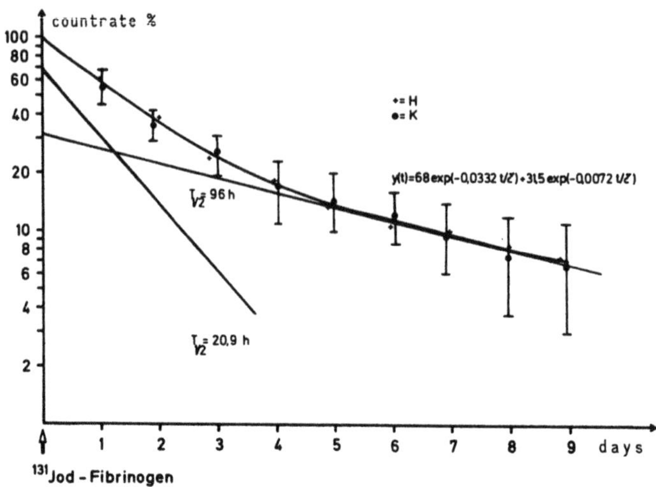

Fig. 4.3:
Kinetics of I-131 fibrinogen after measurement over heart (H) and head (K), semi - logarithmic. Fit with biexponential expression, using the curve peeling method. Representation of the two components

4.2 Radionuclide Angiocardiography

An application of engymetry for the assessment of short-term processes is to be found in first-pass radionuclide angiocardiography (88,93,95). With first-pass techniques using radioactive blood volume and blood flow indicators, hemodynamic measurements are possible regarding:

- cardiac output
- transit times (mean, minimal)
- pulmonary blood volume
- ejection and filling rates
- ejection fraction
- end-systolic and end-diastolic volume
- stroke volume
- shunt quantification

The instrumental approach is either through imaging with the gamma-camera and ROI-techniques (regions of interest) or non-imaging with single probes (31,69,95,189,191,200,209). Fig. 4.4 shows first-pass precordial curves after the intravenous bolus injection of 4 mCi H_2 O-15 as one example of the applicatior of MIESSY. The radiation detection subsystem used is the double radionuclide detector of Fig. 2.7. Its placement over the left lung during another measurement for left-to-right shunt detection is shown with the X-ray chest of Fig. 4.8. The passage of the indicator bolus through the right and left heart is easily recognizable. Temporal and spatial resolution in this example is not sufficient to distinguish single heartbeats. The preliminary engymetric determinations of the common circulation parameters mentioned above with Tc-99m are in agreement with corresponding comparative measurements with the gamma-camera.

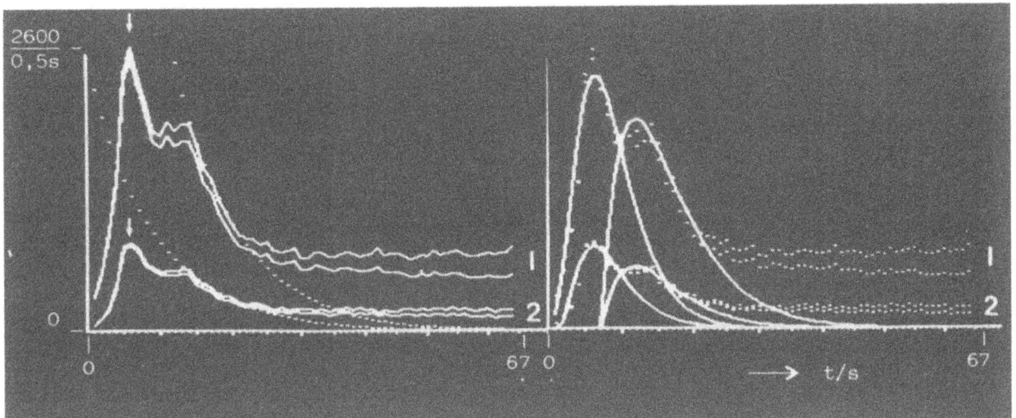

Fig. 4.4:
Radionuclide angiocardiography with 4 mCi H_2 O-15 and precordial GM tubes arrangement for double-radionuclide measurement after Figs. 2.6-2.8. Count-rates of the 5 GM-tubes in front of (1) and behind lead filter (2). The first peak corresponds to the passage through the right heart (arrow) and the second through the left. The upper curve is decay-corrected in each case. Monoexponential fit of left heart, washout (left). Fit of dextro- and laevocardial phases with gamma-variate (right) (without subtraction) (158).
Sampling interval: 1 sec, counting interval: 0.5 sec, total measurement time: 64 sec

In addition to the precordial counting techniques of first-pass radionuclide angiocardiography there is another potent cardiovascular Nuclear Medicine procedure: the ECG-gated equilibrium blood pool method. Here red blood cells or plasma proteins which cannot leave the vascular system are labeled with radioactive tracers (168). Using the R-wave of the ECG as a physiological trigger, many heart cycles are added synchronously. This feature, controlling the acquisition by ECG-gating, has not yet been implemented with MIESSY. As a preparation for such engymetric measurements, experience with a cardiac scintillation probe technique for determining the ejection fraction and other hemodynamic parameters was gathered by using the Nuclear Stethoscope (31,95,191,200,201,209). This mobile instrument, which is called portable although the probe is fixed to a probe arm on a small wheeled vehicle containing microprocessor, CRT-display, and operator's console, and which depends on external electric power supply, has been proved useful in a variety of clinical and research applications for cardiac monitoring. These include rehabilitation programs, surgical applications, pacemaker programming, evaluation of interventions such as drugs, exercise, hand grip, cold pressor response, and continuous monitoring during anesthesia.

Material and Method

Details concerning the method of application and clinical use of the single probe are to be found in (31,95,191,200,201,209). In addition, we attached a light source to the scintillation probe of the Nuclear Stethoscope so that we could control the field of view of the crystal which is in a suspended position above the chest. Any changes in the position of the patient during measurement have to be carefully avoided. Control is facilitated by a point of light marked on the chest wall (108).

57 patients were examined with the single probe immediately after angiocardiography and/or ECG-gated equilibrium blood pool scintigraphy (108). Three groups A, B, C were formed:

A: all patients
B: excluding patients with dyskinetic wall motion
C: only patients with verified dyskinesis

Results and Discussion

There was good reproducibility with regard to positioning. With 28 patients the determination of the ejection fraction (EF) was carried out twice without altering the position of the probe. With 16 patients the determination of EF was also carried out twice, but after repositioning the probe (r=0.99, N=28 and r=0.98, N=16) (108).

Correlation of ejection fraction from the Nuclear Stethoscope with

ECG-gated blood pool scintigraphy	group A	r=0.87	N=27	p<0.001
	group B	r=0.87	N=19	p<0.001
	group C	r=0.54	N= 8	p=0.085
angiocardio-graphy	group A	r=0.73	N=35	p<0.001
	group B	r=0.76	N=21	p<0.005
	group C	r=0.65	N=18	p<0.005

Table 4.2:
Comparison of the ejection fraction determined by different methods (108)

Table 4.2 includes the results of the measurements with the single probe after correlation with the two reference methods (invasive angiocardiography, non-invasive ECG-gated equilibrium blood pool scintigraphy). It shows that the measurement accuracy of the single probe is restricted in cases of severe regional wall motion abnormalities, such as aneurysms, as well as of hyperkinetic and akinetic abnormalities.

The firm attachment of a number of single MIESSY probes to the chest wall could possibly eliminate this disadvantage. Fig. 4.5 illustrates the dependence of the EF determined with the Nuclear Stethoscope on the position of the probe (108). The detector does not touch the thorax wall.

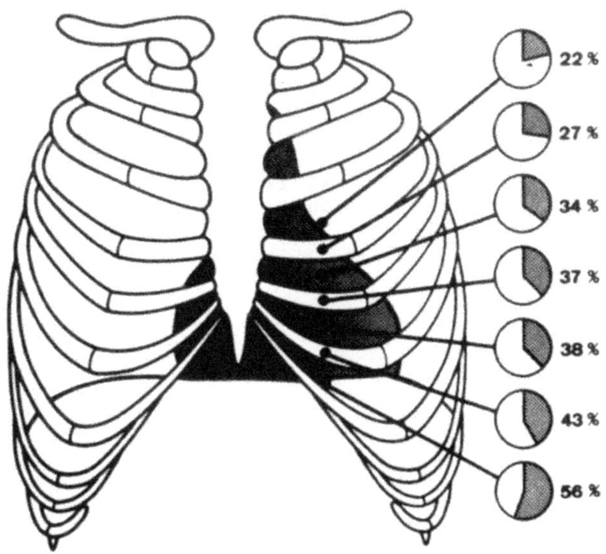

Fig. 4.5:
Ejection fraction (%) dependent on detector position (108)

Conclusions

These preliminary studies and other clinical work (31,88,95,191,201,209) show that reproducible results can be obtained with the single probe technique. For examinations such as these it is MIESSY that is really portable because of its low weight and its own energy supply. In contrast to the situation with the Nuclear Stethoscope the patient can move freely with the attached measurement system. Engymetric examinations are possible without disturbing the monitoring of patients by other means in intensive care units.

However, in contrast to the established Nuclear Stethoscope, additions to the system, such as ECG-triggering and further clinical experience will be necessary (88,93) before MIESSY can be used more extensively in clinical cardiology. In particular, the question must be examined of whether the poor correlation of the EF with the reference methods found especially in the critically ill of group C (Table 4.2) can be improved through the attachment over the heart region of a number of miniaturized radiation detectors, in the manner of a real portable gamma camera. For serial studies of the patients, e.g. after heart attacks, the dependence of the EF on the detector position (Fig. 4.5) would then probably provide better measurement results.

4.2.1 RIGHT-TO-LEFT SHUNTS

Another clinical application of engymetry in Nuclear Medicine detected and estimated intracardiac right-to-left shunts in children, comparing countrates from In-113m labeled microspheres over head, kidneys and lungs after intravenous injection. In existing intracardiac right-to-left shunts particles bypass the pulmonary circulation. They are trapped by systemic embolism and lead to scintigraphic visualisation, mainly of the kidneys and brain (77,78,192). The engymetric examinations took place during and after routine lung scanning.

The portable scaler-timer of Fig. 2.5 was employed for this. Useful hints at the pulmonary or cardiac origin of cyanosis in children can be obtained in this way, for example immediately after birth. Fig. 4.6 shows a comparison of results produced by the large stationary gamma camera with those of engymetry.

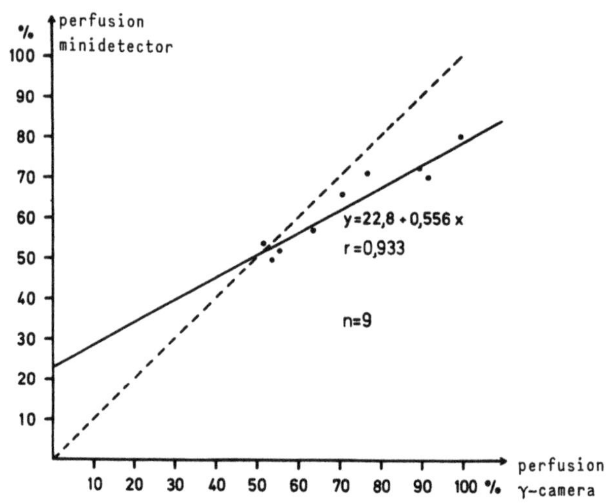

Fig. 4.6:
Relative perfusion of the right lung in 9 children (6 months - 5 years) with intracardiac right-to-left shunts. Comparison between lung imaging with computer processing and engymetric measurements

Although the correlation of relative lung perfusion between gamma camera and minidetector seems high in this small group of children these are only preliminary results. The clinical usefulness remains to be determined.

4.2.2 LEFT-TO-RIGHT SHUNTS

Left-to-right shunts can be quantified after the inhalation of CO_2-15 and registration of time-activity-curves during washout over the lungs (43,137,194,204,205). If a left-to-right shunt is present, then during washout of the immediately labeled venous pulmonary blood water a sudden increase of countrates over the lungs occurs because of the left-to-right shunt flow. The immediate labeling of the pulmonary venous blood water results from the conversion of the diffused CO_2 -15 by carbonic anhydrase to H_2CO_3 dissociating to H_2O (204). Fig. 4.7 shows individual and added curves of three GM detectors over right lung and heart. The positioning of the individual GM detectors on the chest can be seen in Fig. 4.8.

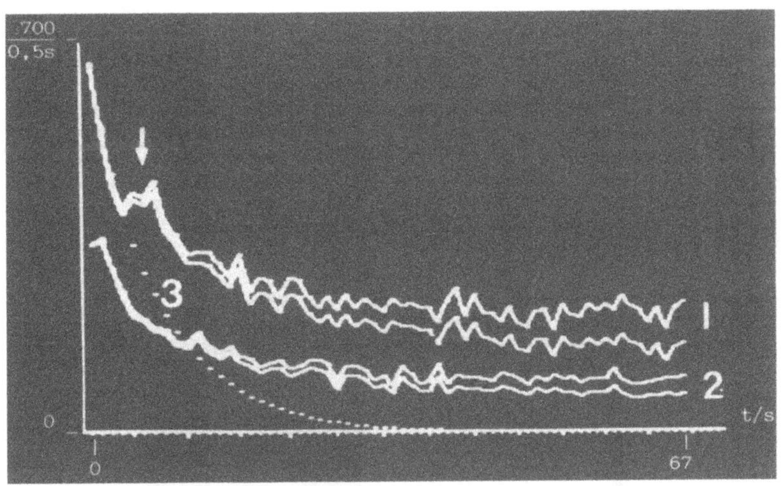

Fig. 4.7:
Left-to-right shunt measurement after bolus inhalation of 5 mCi CO_2 -15. Added curves of two GM detectors over right lung (1) with shunt flow (arrow). Heart curve from one detector (2). In each case the upper curve is the decay corrected curve of the one beneath it. Monoexponential fit of the washout phase (3) for shunt calculation after WATSON (204,205).
Sampling interval: 1 sec, counting interval: 0.5 sec, total measurement time: 64 sec

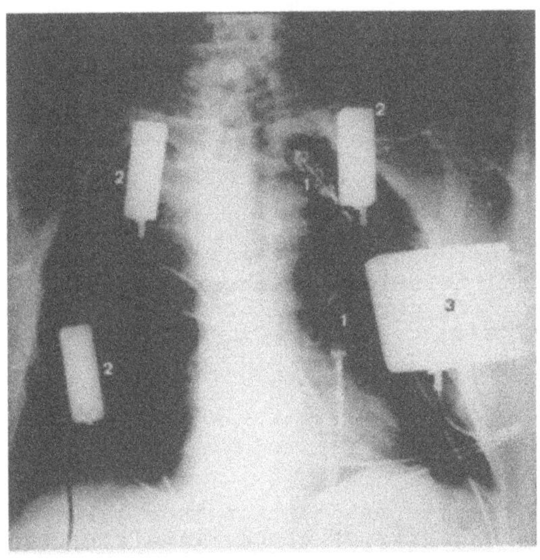

Fig. 4.8:
Position of GM detectors around the chest in X-ray photograph. Not collimated (1), collimated (2), double nuclide detector (3) (see Figs. 2.6 - 2.8)

Results and Discussion

The small peak during lung washout can be clearly recognized (Fig. 4.7). Curve analysis with DISYA produces a left-to-right shunt of Qp/Qs =2.2. Fig. 4.9 shows the comparable time-activity-histograms from the right lung and heart with the ROI technique after acquisition of data, at the same time, with an imaging emission computerized tomography system (positron camera with dual opposite multicrystal heads, Model 4200, Cyclotron Corporation). The same flow ratio is calculated with the imaging device. It is also in agreement with the result of the dye dilution analysis.

After the intravenous bolus injection of 99m-TcO_4^-, the intracardiac left-to-right shunt determination can also be carried out engymetrically after curve fitting with DISYA by means of gamma variates (151).

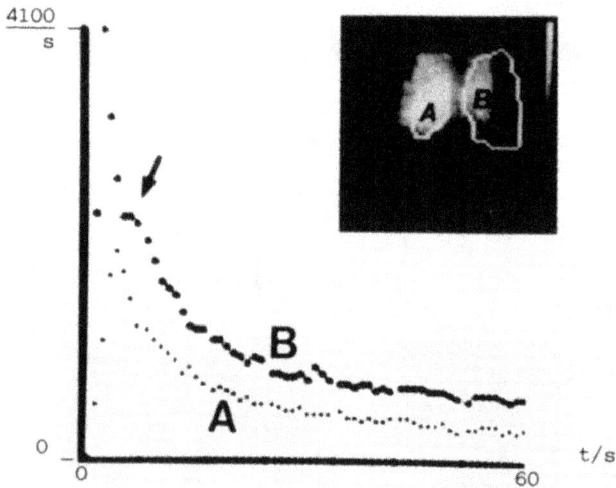

Fig. 4.9:
Simultaneous measurement as in Figs. 4.7, 4.8 with positron camera and ROI-technique. Right: position of ROI over heart (A) and right lung (B) in longitudinal emission tomogram. Below: corresponding time activity histograms (not corrected for decay). Arrow: peak from shunt flow. Frame rate: 1/sec

4.3 Chronic venous insufficiency

With physiological changes of position from lying to sitting, standing or walking there are shifts of blood into the leg vein system. The normal pressure-dependent venous capacity, i.e. the blood volume in the leg veins increases by 350 ml on average (217). Arterio-venous pressure gradient, calf muscle pump, ankle joint pump and the valves of deep and superficial veins direct the blood flow back to the heart, assisted by a complex system of perforating one-way valves in the calf muscle pump. This normal return of blood is disturbed in the case of chronic venous insufficiency and results in the increased filtration of edema into the tissue (70,175,216,217).

In order to objectify the extent of edema in the postthrombotic syndrome as well as the effectiveness of compression stockings on blood volume and edema within extremities, the dynamics of extracellular and intravascular fluid volumes can be measured engymetrically (156,158). Because of the easy transportability of MIESSY for the first time tests can be carried out continuously without telemetric radio transmission during various physiologic maneuvers, in a lying, sitting, standing and walking position.

Material and Method

The measurements were performed on 5 normal and 14 postthrombotic legs. 30 µCi Br-82 were used as radioindicator for the extracellular compartment, and 1 mCi Tc-99m in vivo labeled red blood cells for the intravascular compartment (124,142,156,158). Br-82 and Tc-99m are injected intravenously 24 hours and 30 minutes respectively before the measurement. The discrimination of the two radionuclides is carried out by means of the GM detector arrangements for double nuclide measurements after Fig. 2.8. The countrates in the Tc-99m channel are corrected with regard to Br-82 according to section 2.1.1.

It has not yet been determined to what extent the measured countrates N (t) (eq. 2.1) change in a non-linear manner with the radioactively labeled extracellular and intravascular fluid volume contents. For this reason the data are calculated as a volume index. In addition, questions concerning extravasation of the Tc-99m after the in vivo labeling of the red blood cells and intracellular Br-82 losses are not taken into consideration (124,142).

Results

Fig. 4.10 demonstrates the result of a double radionuclide measurement with Br-82 and Tc-99m. One of the GM-counter arrangements (Fig. 2.8) was attached to the right and one to the left calf of a patient with postthrombic syndrome of the left side. Signals were registered continuously before, during and after the interventions. After changes in the position from lying (a) to walking (b) the countrates rise steeply in the Tc-99m channels in both legs, dependent on the increasing blood volume in the lower leg. This is more prominent in the left than in the right leg. In the Br-82 channel, corresponding to the extracellular fluid volume, there is at first a slow continuous increase in the left leg (b), and then, during a break in the walking, compared with Tc-99m (intravascular index), an overproportional increase in both sides. After compression stockings have been put on (f) and after walking again (g), the former maxima (b,d) are no longer reached. The original values are restored after the patient is in a lying position (h) again.

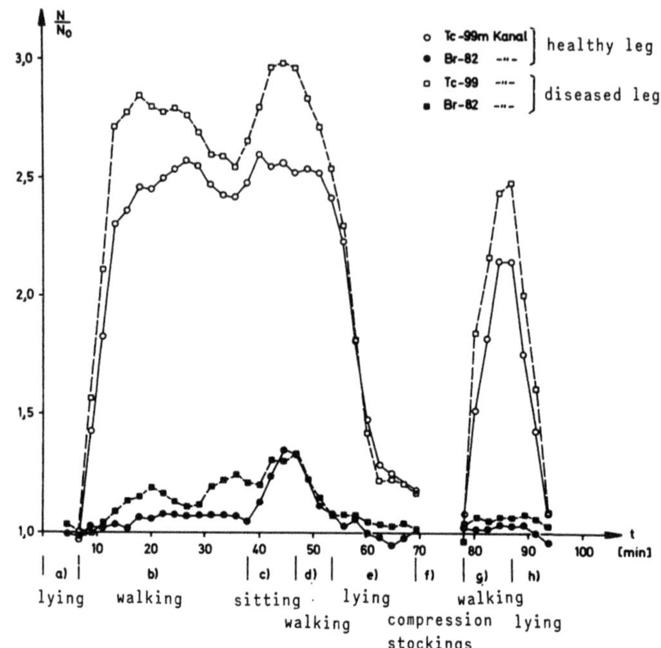

Fig. 4.10:
Engymetric double radionuclide measurement (Tc-99m, Br-82) on both calves with a postthrombotic syndrome in the left. Interventions: lying, sitting, standing, walking. Countrates decay - corrected and normalized to original values in lying position.
Sampling interval: 2.2 min, counting interval: 1.1 min, total measurement time: 1.6 hours

Results of measurements on 5 healthy legs with and without a compression stocking (class III) are summarized in Fig. 4.11. Fig. 4.12 shows the corresponding results of measurements on 14 legs with a postthrombotic syndrome.

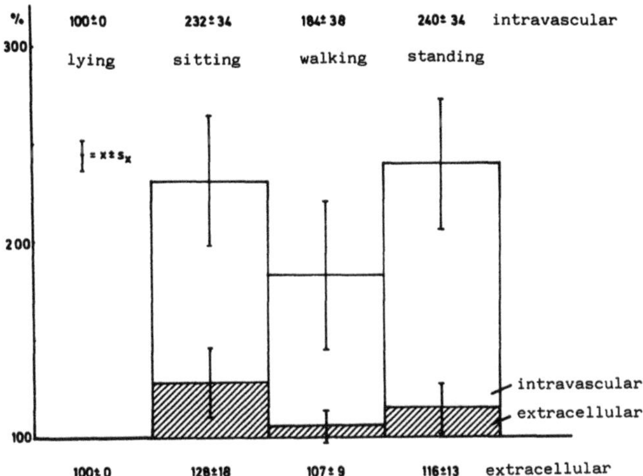

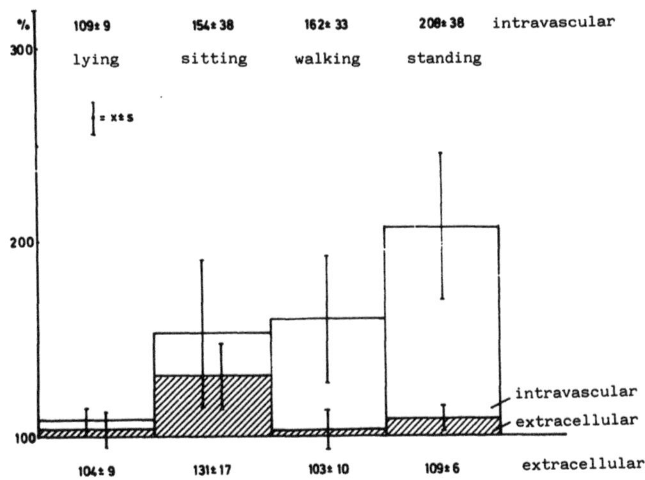

Fig. 4.11:
Simultaneous change of intravascular blood volume and extracellular fluid in the healthy leg
Top : without compression, below: with compression stockings

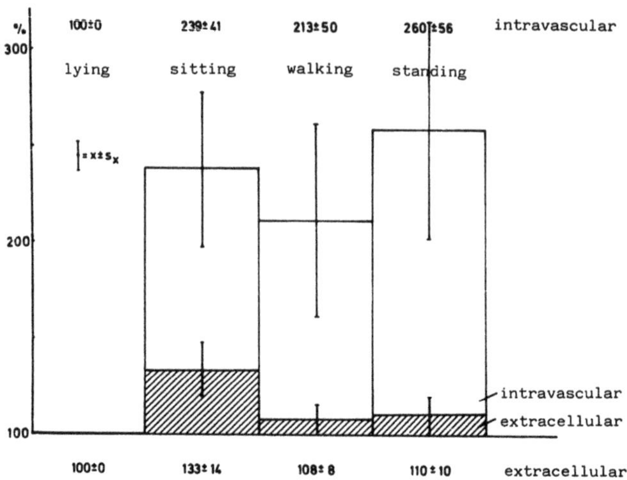

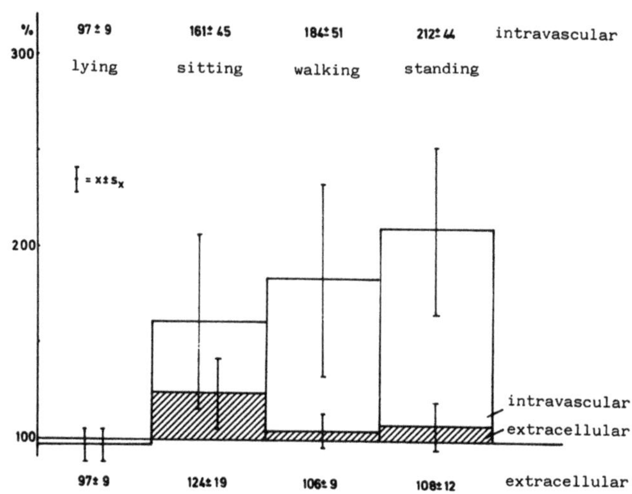

Fig. 4.12:
Simultaneous change of intravascular blood volume and extracellular fluid volume in postthrombotic syndrome
Top: without compression, below: with compression stockings

The number of normal patients (N=5, Fig.4.11) does not seem to be sufficient for statistical comparison. The statistical evaluation (t-test, linear regression) of the results in patients with a postthrombotic syndrome demonstrates:

1. Comparison of the intravascular and extracellular volume index after change of position with and without compression:

		Intravascular	Extracellular
sitting	(N=12)	$p<0.0005$	n.s
standing	(N= 9)	$p<0.001$	n.s
walking	(N=14)	$p<0.0005$	n.s

   There is a significant alteration of intravascular volume from the state without compression to that with compression. The volume index falls up to 33% during sitting, to 19% during standing and to 14% during walking. The differences in the two fluid volume compartments between sitting and standing (N=9; $p<0.0005$) and between sitting and walking (N=13; $p<0.0005$) are also significant.

2. The differences between intravascular and extracellular volume change are significant between sitting and standing without compression, both at $p<0.005$ (N=14). Under compression only the extracellular fluid volume changes significantly between sitting and standing (N=13; $p<0.0001$), while the intravascular change of volume, on the other hand, is not significant (n.s.).

3. In a comparison of the intravascular and extracellular volume index, alterations after a change of position provide the following results in linear regression:

		Without compression	With compression
sitting	(N=14)	$r=0.13$	$r=0.39$
standing	(N= 9)	$r=0.79$ ($p<0.01$)	$r=0.6$
walking	(N=14)	$r=0.45$	$r=0.34$

Discussion

Tests on venous hemodynamics with radioindicators are described in the literature (74,134,184). The methods used till now have been mechanically complicated tilting and rotating bed apparatuses which are electronically controlled, and into which the patient is securely strapped (74,184).

Continuous Nuclear Medical measurements of venous hemodynamics during physiological actions (lying, sitting, standing, walking) without limitations to the patient's mobility have been unknown till now. Reference methods not employing Nuclear Medicine procedures, for example phlebography or plethysmography, seem to be only slightly suitable for the purpose of distinguishing the individual changes in the intravascular and extracellular fluid compartments of the lower extremities simultaneously, continously, and without adversely affecting the patient while lying, sitting, standing or walking.

The results described here must be regarded as preliminary because of the lack of reference and the small number of cases. However, they elucidate the clinical use of MIESSY for estimating quantitatively the effect of compression stockings on the intravascular and extracellular volumes in the postthrombotic syndrome and after physiological changes of position.

In the relatively short measurement time during individual physiological maneuvers, the compression stocking has a significant effect in reducing the blood volume of the lower leg during sitting, and the smallest effect during walking (70,175,217), but still at least an additional 14%. The compression stocking does not significantly reduce the extracellular volume, as the measurement time (approx. 15 min) may be too short, although rapid changes in the extracellular volume index can be observed in the change from sitting to walking (Figs. 4.10 - 4.12).

The clear rise in the extracellular volume index during sitting may be caused by the alteration of flow in the lymphatic system and of the blood reflux in the groin (70,175,217). The change in the volume indices occurs in the same direction in the normal and pathological vein system. Quantitative differences cannot be found between the normal patients tested and those with the postthrombotic syndrome as regards their volume indices under compression.

Blood volume index and extracellular volume index only correlate during standing without compression, possibly as a result of the short measurement time.

Further measurements are necessary for a better understanding of the pathophysiology of the postthrombotic syndrome and the effect of compression therapy on this disease. The preliminary results with MIESSY seem to demonstrate that the use of this method is of high interest.

4.4 Compartment Syndrome

Together with their blood vessels and nerves, the muscle groups of the extremities lie in firm fascias and form functional units, so-called compartments. In the case of the compartment syndrome, muscular microcirculatory disturbances with increasing functional losses occur within these compartments (60,130,131,135). The highly swollen muscles have no possibility of expanding. If not treated, this often results in muscle necrosis (60,118). The problem of this illness lies in the difficulty of making an early diagnosis. There is a danger of not recognizing a developing compartment syndrome in the cases where the significance of ischemia-induced pain is not recognized, or where it is concealed by the uncontrolled prescription of analgetics. Making the diagnosis is problematic, particularly with seriously injured or unconscious patients, since the subjective criteria are missing here. In order to objectify the pressure rise in a fascial loge, the pressure measurement is carried out using the needle and wick catheter method (59,131,135).

Method

Since pressure measurement is not always possible because, for example, bandages are in the way, a new, non-invasive, engymetric method for quantifying posttraumatic edema was examined in an animal model experiment (59). In order to characterize the extent and kinetics of edemas of the extremities, the time course of the radioactive bromide (Br-82) as a tracer of the extracellular fluid volume was measured in comparison to the healthy extremity (59,124). 50 male wistar rats were subjected to a standardized soft tissue trauma under a Ketanest - Rompun narcosis after each animal had been given 10 µCi Br-82 intraperitoneally. Two groups were formed, each containing 25 animals. The first group was subjected to a direct contusion of the flexor muscles of the rear leg for 30 minutes. In the second group a tourniquet was applied for 2 hours. Parallel to the activity measurement, the interstitial pressure in the flexors was registered via a wick catheter by means of a Statham element (59).

Results

Neither in group 1 nor in group 2 was it possible with the wick catheter in the traumatized section of the extremity to objectify any significant increase of the interstitial pressure when compared with the control extremity of the other side (Fig. 4.13). In both groups countrates of Br-82 over time run parallel to the clinical diagnosis (Fig. 4.13).

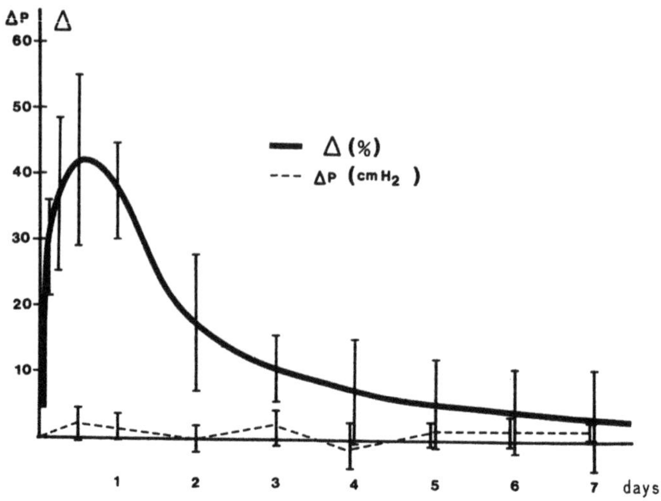

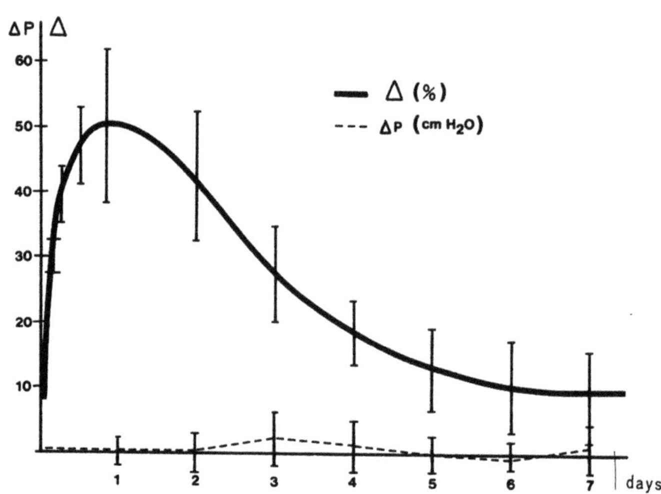

Fig. 4.13:
Top : graph of the relative change of Br-82 countrates (%) in comparison with intramuscular pressure differences ΔP(cm H_2O) between healthy and damaged rear leg of the rat (N=25) after muscle cortusion (group 1) (59).
Below: comparison of the relative change of Br-82 countrates (%) with intramuscular pressure differences ΔP(cm H_2O) between healthy and damaged rear leg of the rat (N=25) after loosening of the tourniquet after two hours (group 2) (59)

With a traumatized patient after the reimplantation of the lower left leg it was possible to register the postoperative Br-82 kinetics symmetrically with 4 GM detectors, two each on the healthy and affected lower leg. In spite of the prophylactic fasciotomy of all 4 loges after the reimplantation edema increases in the replanted section of the limb. After skin relaxation and the splitting of the ligamentum transversum cruris the edema was reduced at first by 20%. During the following days a rebound compartment syndrome arose, and this was registered engymetrically at a very early stage (Fig. 4.14) (130,158).

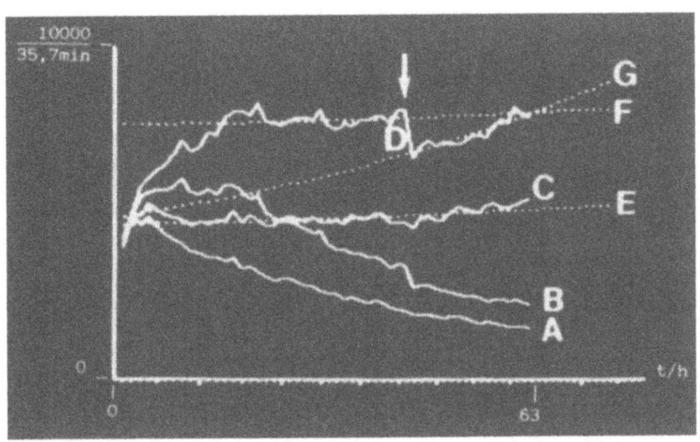

Fig. 4.14:
Br-82 kinetics after the reimplantation of a lower leg and operative relief (25 µCi Br-82 i.v.). Countrates as the sum of the signals from two detectors over the healthy lower leg (A) and two over the affected one (B). After decay correction (C,D) fit by means of slowly rising exponential functions (E,F). Relief by surgery (arrow). Subsequent recurrence with monoexponential rise (G).
Sampling interval: 71.5 min, counting interval: 35.7 min, total measurements time: 63 hours

Discussion

In the tests on animals Br-82 proved to be a sensitive indicator of the course of a posttraumatic edema. Both with the tourniquet trauma and after direct muscle contusion it was possible to estimate quantitatively changes in the extracellular fluid volume in a way that could be reproduced (59).

Circulatory disorders of the muscles after ischemia or contusion seem to be documented engymetrically at an earlier stage and more sensitively with the Br-82 tracer method than with traditional measuring methods. An additional advantage is that this is a non-invasive technique which can even be applied when the extremities are held still in a plaster dressing. Measurements can easily be carried out in the intensive care unit. Further experience must be gained before the measurement values can be interpreted pathophysiologically and the clinical consequences arived at.

4.5 Intraoperative blood distribution changes

Within the framework of a study aimed at improving prophylactic measures against thrombosis after neurosurgery on the spine, engymetry was used in 21 patients to find unexpectedly large intravascular fluid volume shifts dependent on the posture during the operation. With the Virchow trias (stasis, hypercoagulability, endothelium changes) recognized as essential for the development of a thrombus, and with the assumptions that postoperative deep vein thromboses of the leg already start intraoperatively (84,115,197), an increased risk of thrombosis with neurosurgery in the knee-chest position was suspected. In order to confirm this suspicion, an investigatory study was begun with the aim of:

1. determining the extent of the intraoperative fluid volume shifts with Br-82 as the tracer for the extracellular and with Tc-99m in vivo labeled red blood cells as the tracer for the intravascular compartment (124,142)
2. demonstrating the development of the intraoperative thromboses with I-131 fibrinogen and autologous platelets labeled with In-111 oxine (81).

Material and Method

23 patients were examined before, during and after their operation. In 19 cases the surgical intervention on the spine took place in the knee-chest position, in two cases while sitting and in two in the prone jackknife position. The engymetric registration of the time activity curves took place continuously and simultaneously through at least 4 (max. 12) measuring points on the body of the patient. These were usually situated on both sides of the lower extremities. In 7 cases measurements were made additionally over the heart, on the upper arm and over the spleen. The radioindicators were in vivo labeled erythrocytes, Br-82, I-131 fibrinogen and autologous platelets labeled with In-111 oxine in dosages of between 20 and 100 µCi. Double radionuclide measurements of Tc-99m together with Br-82 took place in 9 cases using GM detectors arranged as in Figs. 2.7, 2.8.

Results

As an example of intraoperative engymetric data acquisition Fig. 4.15 shows blood volume shifts before, during and after a lumbar disc operation with the patient in the knee-chest position. One collimated GM detector was localized above the heart region and one on the left upper arm. A double radionuclide detector after Fig. 2.8 lay on the right lower leg. Because of regional blood volume shifts during the preoperative moving of the patient, Br-82 and Tc-99m countrates at first decline in the lower leg and rise synchronously in the upper arm. Above the heart region there is a preoperative drop in the countrate. An infusion (500 ml) is assumed to be the reason for this. After the final posture has been assumed, countrates in the lower leg rise continuously. During the operation (1.8 hours) they drop in the upper arm to constant values. Subsequently the blood shifts are correspondingly reversed.

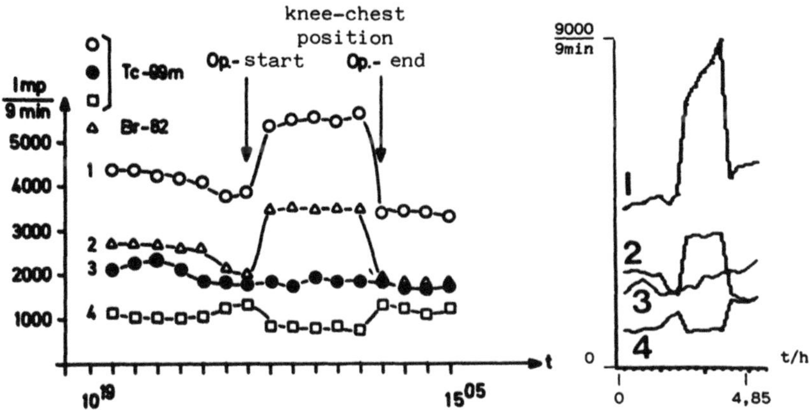

Fig. 4.15:
Intraoperative double radionuclide measurement (18 µCi Tc-99m, 25 µCi Br-82) for demonstration of fluid volume shifts.
Left: Tc-99m countrates at the lower leg (1), precordial (3), at the upper arm (4). Br-82 registration (2) at the lower leg as (1) (not decay corrected)
Right: decay corrected original engygrams
Sampling interval: 18 min, counting period: 9 min, total measurement time: 4.8 hrs

Fig. 4.16 shows a different engymetric registration before, during and after operation, using 50 µCi I-131 fibrinogen. 4 GM detectors after Fig. 2.2,? lay proximally and distal-femorally and tibially. All detectors show an increase in countrates amounting to over 100% during surgery in the knee-chest position, the largest being proximal-femoral ones.

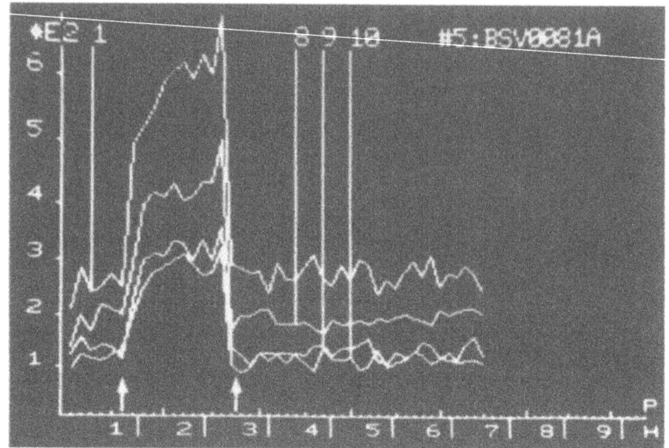

Fig. 4.16:
Engymetric intraoperative and postoperative activity registration over 6.5 hours (H) during an operation (between arrows) in knee-chest position (50 µCi I-131 fibrinogen). Detector positions (GM counters): proximal-femoral (1), distal-femoral (8), proximal-tibial (9), distal-tibial (10).
Sampling interval: 9 min, counting period: 4.5 min, total measurement time: 6.5 hrs

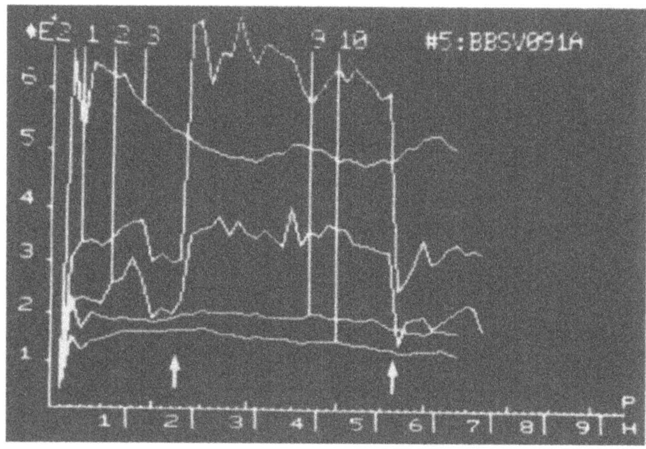

Fig. 4.17:
Engymetric intraoperative activity registration over 7 hours (H) during an operation (between arrows) with patient seated (60 µCi I-131 fibrinogen). Detector positions (GM counters): proximal-femoral (1), distal-femoral (2), proximal-femoral (9), distal-tibial (10), precordial (3).
Sampling interval: 18 min, counting period: 9 min, total measurement time: 7 hrs

Of the two patients with a cervical vertebra operation in a sitting position one measurement is shown in Fig. 4.17 after the application of 60 µCi I-131 fibrinogen. In this example there are proximal-femoral and distal-femoral intraoperative countrate increases, while the activity reduces precordially. The countrates over the lower legs, which in this position are situated at the same height as the diaphragm, remain constant. As a result of the finding of the unexpectedly high countrate increases above the legs during an operation in the knee-chest position and because of an assumed increased risk of thrombosis, lumbar disc operations were performed on two patients in the prone jackknife position. Fig. 4.18 shows as an example a measurement result with autologous platelets labeled with 90 µCi In-111 oxine. The labeling was carried out with reference to the procedure by GOODWIN et al (81). The countrates remain constant above the lower extremities during the four-hour operation.

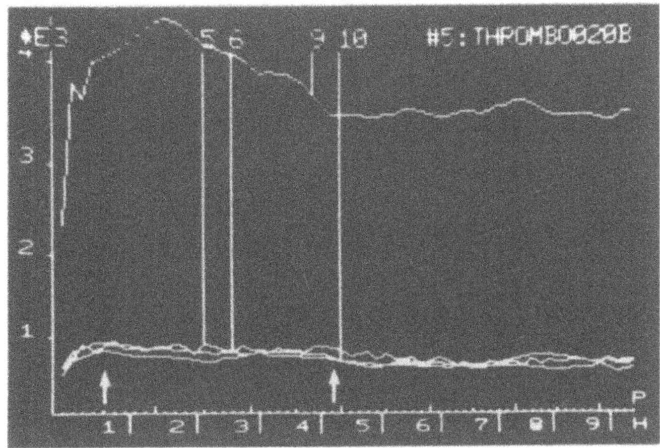

Fig. 4.18:
Engymetric intraoperative activity registration over 9 hours (H) in an operation (between arrows) with the patient in prone jackknife position (autologous thrombocytes labeled with 90 µCi In-111 oxine). Detector positions (GM counters): above calf right (5), above calf left (6), spleen (9), femoral left (10).
Sampling interval: 9 min, counting period: 4.5 min, total measurement time: 9.6 hrs

Among the 23 patients examined there was only one case with a thrombosis, a pelvic thrombosis, between the first and second day after the operation. Fig. 4.19 shows the femoral and tibial countrates registered with this patient.

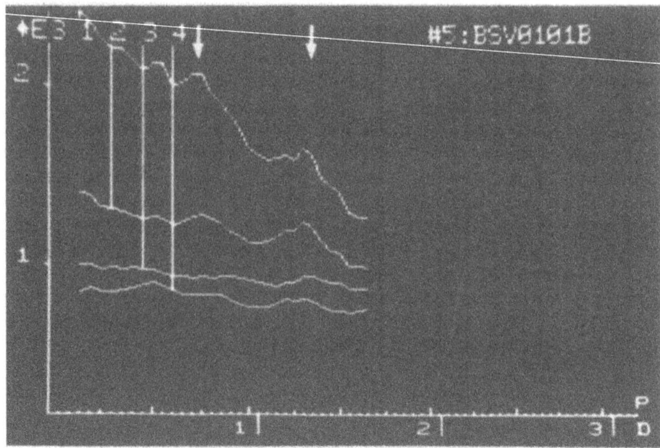

Fig. 4.19:
Engymetric postoperative activity registration over 1.6 days (D) after the operation in knee-chest position (60 μCi I-131 fibrinogen). Detector positions (GM counters): proximal-femoral (1), distal-femoral (2), proximal-tibial (3), distal-tibial (4). Discrete countrate increase femorally on second day after operation (arrows).
Sampling interval: 71 min, counting period: 35 min, total measurement time: 1.6 days

Discussion

With the first 23 patients in the current study, all of whom were observed continuously before, during and after the operation using engymetric methods employing I-131 fibrinogen and In-111 labeled platelets, there has so far been no case with a thrombosis commencing during the operation and which it was possible to prove by means of a corresponding countrate increase. With the exception of the pelvic vein thrombosis (Fig. 4.19) on the second day after the operation, there was clinically no reason for suspecting a thrombosis in any of the cases. The slight countrate increase in the case of the pelvic vein thrombosis on the second day after the operation (Fig. 4.19), which was proximal-femoral and distal-femoral, might be explained by a temporary flow obstruction rather than by an increased I-131 fibrinogen deposit in the detector's field of view.

All countrate increases found during the operation dropped to the preoperative level after the operation. They are interpreted as fluid volume increases due to volume shifts. As a result of the limited field of view of the GM counter (Fig. 2.4) and of its particular sensitivity to activity near the detector, however, it cannot be excluded with certainty that pathological tracer accumulations might have been overlooked.

As a preliminary result with clinical consequences, the increase of countrates over both legs in the knee-chest position (19 patients) led in two cases with an increased risk of thrombosis to the prone jackknife position which was not originally planned (Fig. 4.18). After the operation in this posture no thrombosis was suspected with these two patients.

A further preliminary result was that with 4 patients there were regional differences of the engymetrically determined half-life periods of the activity of the thrombocytes labeled with In-111 oxine. The disappearance rate over 2 to 4 days after monoexponential curve fitting varies by up to 48% at measuring points over the heart as representative of the blood, and over the lower extremities.

Above the spleen there are periodic countrate variations with a difference of phase when compared with the variations over the extremities. These findings indicate the possibility of measuring engymetrically for the first time the kinetics of radiopharmaceuticals or labeled blood cells non-invasively, without blood removal. The signals are recorded globally over the heart, representative for the blood, and at the same time regionally, continuously over long periods of time and without the immobilization of the patient under an imaging instrument. Distribution changes can be detected in the whole body.

The engymetric method also enables pharmacologically induced regional redistributions of blood volumes to be registered. SCHOERNER et al. (176) were able to objectify blood shifts of this kind after doses of nitroglycerine to patients with coronary heart disease through measurements beneath a gamma camera with immobilization of the patient.

4.6 Cerebrospinal Fluid Dynamics (Hydrocephalus, Shunts)

In contrast to computed tomography of the brain it is possible through Nuclear Medical cisternography and sequential imaging (after 2,6,24,32,48 hrs) to register cerebrospinal fluid (CSF) dynamics (circulation and drainage) with the use of static scintigrams in different projections (61,64,71,138,139,177). With the ROI technique time-activity-histograms are only possible over relatively short periods of time, so long as the patients can be immobilized (64). Diagnostic measurements similar to the following ones, which are of engymetric nature, were carried out with stationary detector systems, scanners as well as gamma cameras (57,64,139,141,173).

Material and Method

With reference to examinations of this kind, engymetric time-activity-histograms were recorded with 15 patients over the hemispheres, occipitally (high cervically), over the thoracic spine, over the heart, and over the distal lower leg. With these 15 patients cisternography had been routinely carried out previously or simultaneously because of CSF rhinorrhea (9 patients), shunt dysfunctions (4 patients) with hydrocephalus occlusus or communicans and valve closure (2 patients). The application of the radioindicator was by lumbar (11 patients) or occipital (4 patients) injection of 500 µCi In-111-Ca-DTPA.

Results and Discussion

With 9 patients, with whom CSF rhinorrhea could be excluded, there were mean biological half-life periods over the hemispheres of 13 hrs ± 1.6 hrs after lumbar injection. These values are comparable with data given in the literature (141). They are partially lower than the clearance of I-131 labeled human serum albumin (HSA) (127,173).

As a comparison, 4 patients were examined under the same measuring conditions with communicating hydrocephalus after the installation of a ventriculoatrial shunt. Here there was a mean biological half-life period of 3.7 hrs ± 0.5 hrs, which is considerably shorter than before the operation. SANDERS et al. (173) found prolonged half-times of more than 2.5 days for the clearance of I-131 HSA from the subarachnoid space.

With 2 patients suspected of shunt valve dysfunction engymetric measurements were made after intrathecal application via the drainage system situated subcutaneously. The lack of a countrate increase distal to the injection site confirmed the suspected clinical diagnosis, which it was additionally possible to check through operative revision.

Fig. 4.20 shows time-activity-histograms for one of these two patients: a patient on artificial respiration with aqueduct stenosis and posttraumatic hydrocephalus malresorptivus. The measurements were carried out in the neurosurgical intensive care unit.

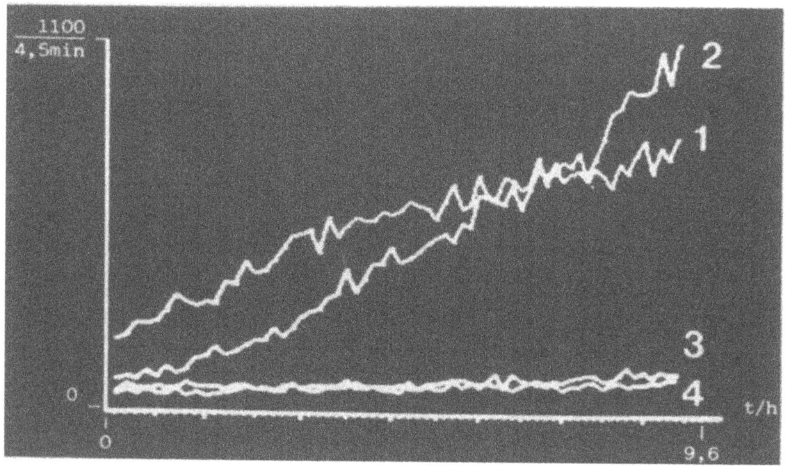

Fig. 4.20:
CSF kinetics in a case of hydrocephalus occlusus (aqueduct stenosis) with ventricular catheter and extracorporeal valve. Activity curves above cisterna magna (1), left hemisphere (2), ventricular catheter (3), collecting vessel (4) (not decay-corrected).
Sampling interval: 9 min, counting period: 4.5 min, total measurement time: 9.6 hrs

It is possible to demonstrate the aqueduct stenosis through the lack of a countrate increase over the extracorporeal ventricular drain. This was additionally confirmed by means of ventriculography. The activity increase is delayed over the cisterna magna and left hemisphere.

In contrast to the situation with engymetry, it is precisely with patients in intensive care or on artificial respiration with whom it is difficult to carry out the method by OTTO et al. (138) for the function control of ventriculoatrial and ventriculoperitoneal shunts using stationary equipment.

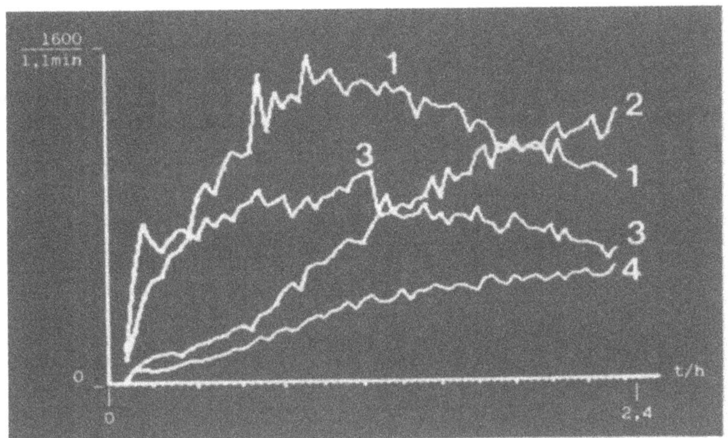

Fig. 4.21:
CSF kinetics in a case of hydrocephalus communicans with ventriculo-atrial shunt (normal pressure). Activity curves over cisterna magna (1), left hemisphere (2), retroauricular catheter (3), heart (4) (not decay-corrected).
Sampling interval: 2.2 min, counting period: 1.1 min, total measurement time: 2.4 hrs

Fig. 4.21 demonstrates CSF kinetics with a ventriculoatrial shunt. After intraventricular application of the radioindicator it is possible to calculate CSF clearance from the ventricle, which can be equated with CSF production when no CSF is washed out through the ependymal layer (138).

The diagnosis of CSF rhinorrhea and otorrhea with introduced tampons and accompanying sequential scintigraphy with the gamma-camera could possibly be complemented by miniature detectors in the nasopharyngeal region. In contrast to studies with the camera, the frequent movements made by children do not disturb an engymetric test.

After passage into the blood, the kinetics of the In-111-Ca-DTPA can be additionally surveyed by detectors over the kidneys and over regions representative of the blood level, e.g. for early recognition of peridural injections.

More experience with engymetric measurements of CSF kinetics on patients with different signs of intracranial pathology is necessary, especially regarding the problems of tissue background correction and detector collimation, before detailed statements about the clinical value are possible.

4.6.1 SHUNT FLOW DETERMINATION

Information about CSF kinetics is of particular diagnostic significance for the clinical management of the drained hydrocephalus. Static-morphologically referred data are only of limited use here. Especially after overdrainage or underdrainage because of an implanted shunt system, it is not possible for any conclusions to be drawn from scintigrams concerning the dimensioning of the flow in the drainage systems which are to be corrected. A procedure was thus developed and employed after phantom measurements (Fig. 4.24) on 6 patients for the quantitative determination of the drainage flow in implanted ventriculoatrial and ventriculoperitoneal shunts.

Method

Figs. 2.11 and 4.22 show the principle of the procedure. 200 µCi Tc-99m pertechnetate are injected in 0.1 ml volume into the catheter. At known distances from each other the miniaturized CdTe probes (Figs. 2.9, 2.11) detect the activity in the catheter. A velocity v can be calculated from temporal distances of the maxima of the activity curves, the spatial distances of the small detectors being known (162, 175a). With the cross-section of the catheter $q=1/4\,\pi\,d^2$ (d, diameter) flow equals

$$F = \frac{\pi}{4} d^2 \frac{\Delta s}{\Delta t} \quad (4.1)$$

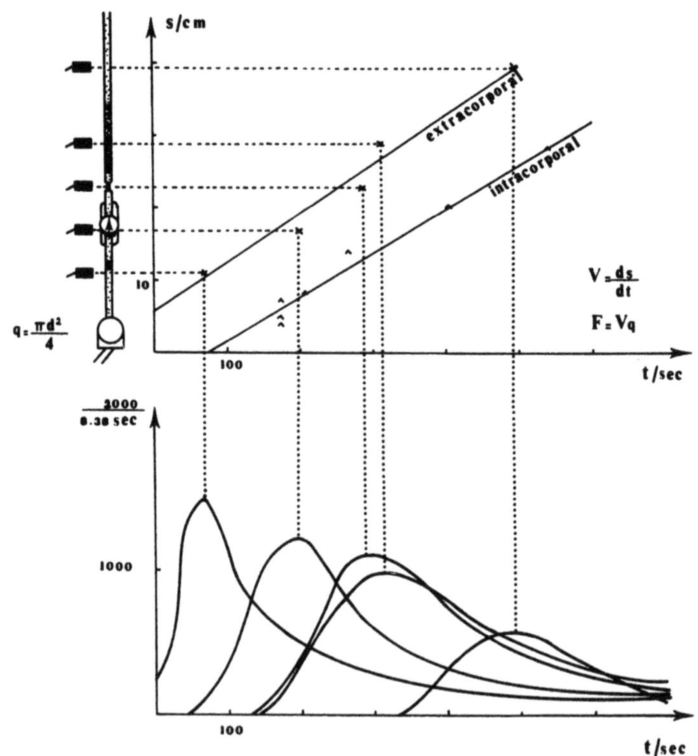

Fig. 4.22:
Principle of shunt flow measurement, distance-time diagram.
Top left: catheter with detectors, top right: results of one extracorporeal and one intracorporeal measurement.
Below: registered time-activity-histograms (schematic) (175a)

Results and discussion

Fig. 4.23 shows the result of phantom measurements with the arrangement according to Figs. 2.11, 4.22.

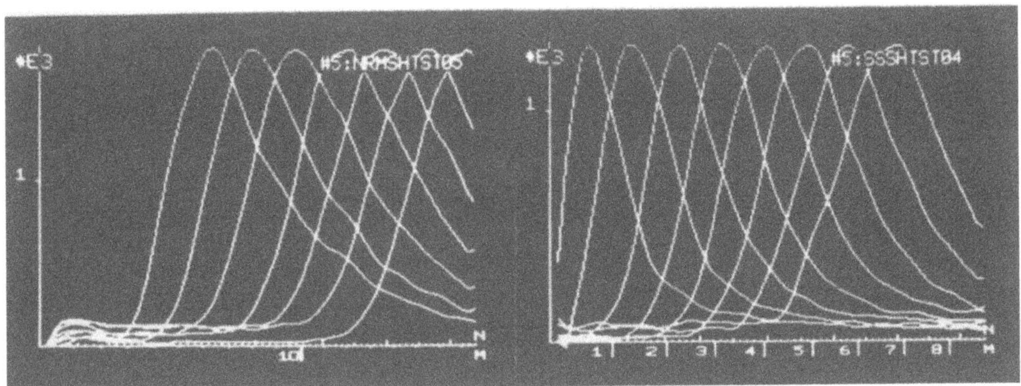

Fig. 4.23:
Registered countrates (see Figs. 2.11, 4.22) with two flows.
Left: 4 ml/h. Sampling interval: 17 sec, counting period: 8 sec.
Right: 8 ml/h. Sampling interval: 8 sec, counting period: 4 sec.
Curves normalized to maximum, abscissa in min (M)

In Fig. 4.24 different flow rates from a precision pump are correlated with the measured and calculated quantities. The differences in the arrival times of the maxima are taken to calculate three flows F between detectors 1-2 (F_1), 2-3 (F_2), and 3-4 (F_3).

The correlation improves with growing distances from the injection site. This might be explained by a transient imbalance of the pressure gradient in the system after injection of the indicator volume proximal to the valve. The results improve with smaller injected volumes (microbolus). CdTe detectors produce sharp peaks in comparison to the broader curves with GM-counters.

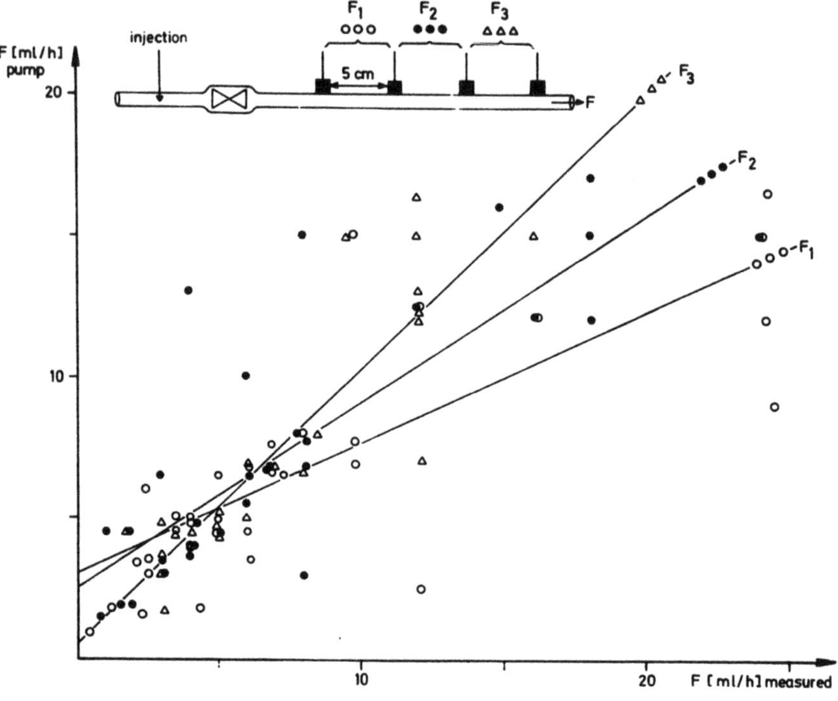

Fig. 4.24:
Correlation of flow rates from phantom experiments according to Figs. 2.11, 4.22. Position of 4 radiation detectors inserted diagrammatically.

F_1 : y = 0.45x + 3.0 ; r = 0.79 ; n = 40
F_2 : y = 0.66x + 2.5 ; r = 0.84 ; n = 38
F_3 : y = 0.97x + 0.6 ; r = 0.87 ; n = 38

Tests which appear to indicate that parameters like minimum transit time, mean transit time and maximum of first derivative on the upslope might be more suitable for the determination of the mean bolus velocity in the drainage system have not yet been completed. The same applies to the cross-correlation technique of Fig. 3.29 (170).

The practical application of the procedure on two patients, an adult and a one week old baby, with subcutaneous catheters and the results are to be found in Figs. 4.25, 4.26.

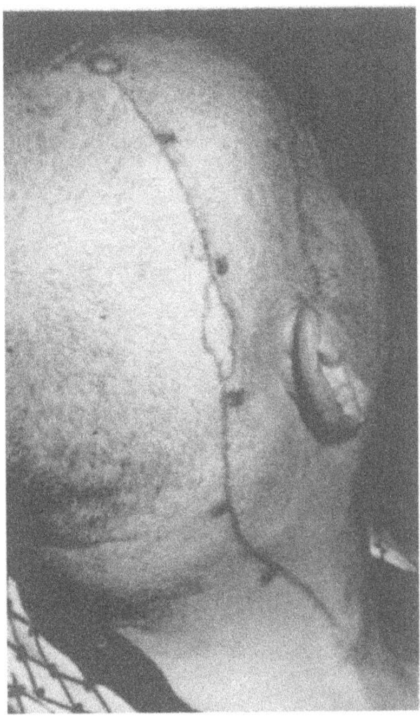

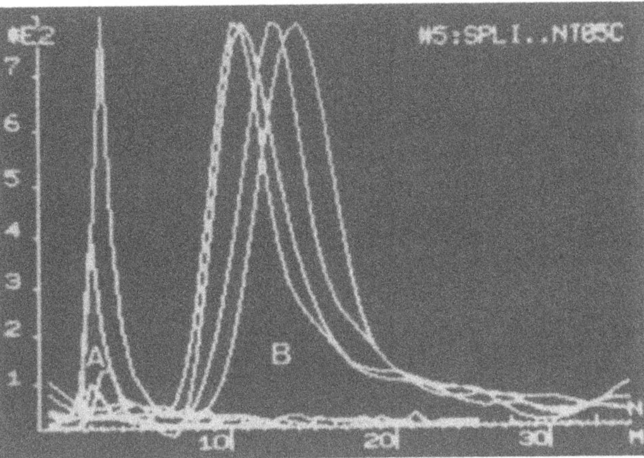

Fig. 4.25:
Ventriculoatrial shunt flow determination in hydrocephalus communicans.
Left: marked subcutaneous course of the catheter, black dots indicating positions of CdTe-detectors
Right: enzymetric time-activity-histograms. A: 4 original curves with different amplitudes from measurement geometry. B: extensions after spline interpolation and normalization to maximum (scaling of abscissa in min (M) does not apply). Shunt flow: 3.2 ml/h.
Sampling interval: 34 sec, counting period: 17 sec

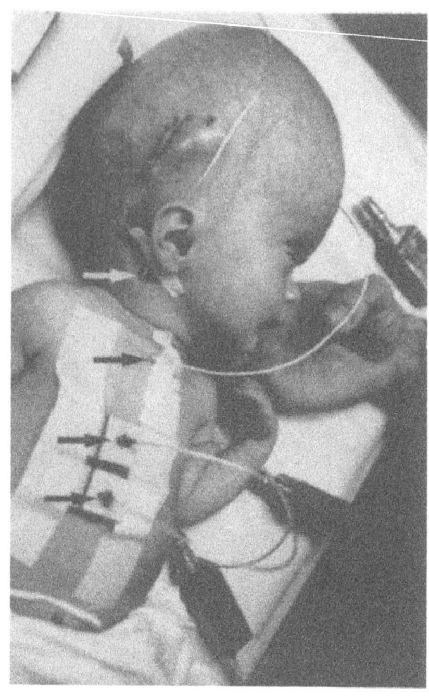

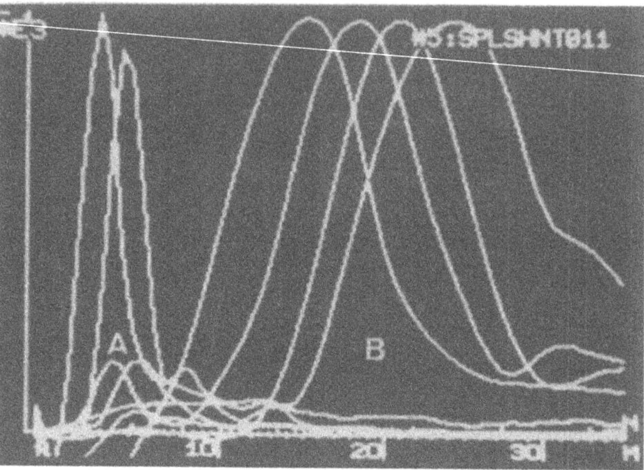

Fig. 4.26:
Ventriculoperitoneal shunt flow determination in hydrocephalus occlusus
Left: position of 4 CdTe detectors (arrows)
Right: engymetric time-activity-histograms. A: 4 original measurement curves with different amplitudes. B: extension after spline interpolation, normalization to maximum (scaling of abscissa in min (M) does not apply). Shunt flow: 4.7 ml/h.
Sampling interval: 34 sec, counting period: 17 sec

KNOETGEN et al. (111) give normal values of between 2.5 and 5 ml/h. On the other hand, the flow index introduced by AKERMAN et al. (6) gives higher values. FUHRMEISTER (75) gives CSF production rates of between 0.15 and 1.55 ml/h.

In the case of the six complication-free patients examined so far, the flow rates vary between 1.7 and 5.3 ml/h. In each case the results are in agreement with the final clinical diagnoses.

The validation of the method is not yet adequate for providing more advanced conclusions. There are indications, however, that an engymetric quantitative determination of the CSF flow in ml/h does provide an early opportunity for the detection of overdrainage or underdrainage after shunt operations as well as the possibility of controlling implanted drainage systems.

The flow measurements described are not continuous for longer time periods. Only the currently labeled CSF shunt flow is calculated dependent on intracranial pressure and the present state of the shunt valve.

4.7 Peripheral Arterial Disease

The peripheral arteriosclerotic disease (PAD) concerns organic changes of the vascular wall, which lead to stenoses or occlusion of the arterial vessel. The disease of the lower extremities is of particular interest since, according to SCHULTE (180), 5% of men between the age of 45 and 65 suffer from it, and at the present time 20,000 leg amputations are carried out anually in the Federal Republic of Germany because of PAD.

Four stages of the disease are defined according to FONTAINE:

I. The disease can be ojectively detected (angiogram, blood vessel sounds), but the patient does not suffer, the disease is completely compensated.

II. Pains occur under walking. At stage

IIa there is relatively good compensation. The length of walking distance is more than 100 m. At stage

IIb the compensation is bad, and the distance is under 100 m.

III. There are pains at rest.

IV. There are necroses with imminent loss of the leg.

Therapeutically, medicamentous therapy or surgical intervention on the blood vessels can be considered. The precise diagnosis with regard to a possible operation is carried out angiographically. The indication to angiography is given from stage IIb to stage IV.

The following complications are described with angiography: contrast medium allergies, with overdosage direct damage to kidney and cerebrum, arteriovenous fistula, intima ablations, as well as thromboembolisms, with which immediate surgical denudation of the blood vessels with thrombectomy becomes necessary. If this is unsuccessful the extremity may be lost. With 13,207 angiographies McAFEE (132) cites 40 cases of death (0.3 %) and 92 (0.7 %) serious, non-lethal incidents. DAVIDSON (55) publishes the same data. Both authors give a frequency of 15 - 20 % for less serious complications, such as temporary restrictions to kidney functions. An even higher risk is described by GUDBJERG (82) for the PAD patient with previously damaged blood vessels.

In addition to angiography there are methods of Nuclear Medicine which are available for measuring the blood supply. These methods were published for the first time in 1949 by KETY (107). After the first results with Na-24 obtained by WALDER (202) in the case of patients with intermittent claudication, the use of Xe-133 became common practice for this examination (30a,52a,58a,119,120,121a,126a). A validation of this method was presented by LASSEN (121) in 1965 through the simultaneous measurement of the blood supply to the muscles with vein occlusion plethysmography, as well as by ALPERT (9) through a comparison of the results of angiography with those of Xe-133 muscle clearance, and by HENNINGES (91) through a comparison between stress oscillography, the ultrasonic Doppler technique and vein occlusion plethysmography.

If the Xe-133 muscle clearance has not been accepted as the standardized routine examination method in the clinic for the diagnosis of PAD this may be because:

1. the technical and financial effort required is relatively high
2. with angiography carried out when PAD is suspected it is possible to guarantee the diagnosis, and it has the advantage that the blood vessel change can be localized precisely.

The development of MIESSY now makes it possible for

1. the necessary technical and financial effort to be considerably restricted, and
2. for the examination to be carried out, not only with stationary machines, but in out-patient departments or directly at the patient's bedside in the ward.

The present examinations are being carried out to answer the question of whether the employment of MIESSY provides a reliable diagnosis, and whether angiography, which is often carried out and is not free of risk, can be replaced for selected cases by Xe-133 muscle clearance. During stage IIa there is no indication yet which justifies an operation, and the complications regarding angiography must not be overlooked.

Method

The method employed in the measurements that have been carried out is as follows:

The patient rests for 5 minutes on the diagnostic couch. Injection of 500 μCi Xe-133 in the m. tibialis anterior, 5-minute measurement of the washout at rest, application of arterial occlusion for 5 minutes, while as many dorsoplantar flexions as possible are performed up to the pain barrier, relaxing of the occlusion and measurement of the maximum blood flow during the following reactive hyperemia.

The time T_m of the maximum blood flow (MBF) is determined in addition to the MBF itself.

Fig. 4.27 shows a measurement result from a patient with unilateral PAD, stage III, as an example of obtaining the blood flow by means of the Xe-133 clearance method. At the same time Fig. 4.27 demonstrates in an exemplary way the result of a dialog session with DISYA (see section 3.3) for determining the blood supply. The results in Fig. 4.27 are obtained after the following interactive actions (the numbers refer to the individual curves in Fig. 4.27):

1. double 7-point smoothing of the original curve (1,2)
2. differentiation of the two smoothed curves (3,4) after spline interpolation with cubic polynomial
3. the first two derivative curves multiplied with (-1) are only raised segmentally for the region of maximum blood supply due to the addition of suitable constants into the positive region of the graph above the measurement curves (5,6)
4. the times of the extrema are determined for both curves (5,6) T_m
5. in the region round these times (±3 measurement points) monoexponential curve fitting (7,8) takes place with parameter

determination

6. this produces the blood flow F in ml/min/100g (d=0.7 diffusion coefficient between muscle and blood) by means of the known relation

$$F = \frac{d \ln 2}{T_{1/2}} \tag{4.2}$$

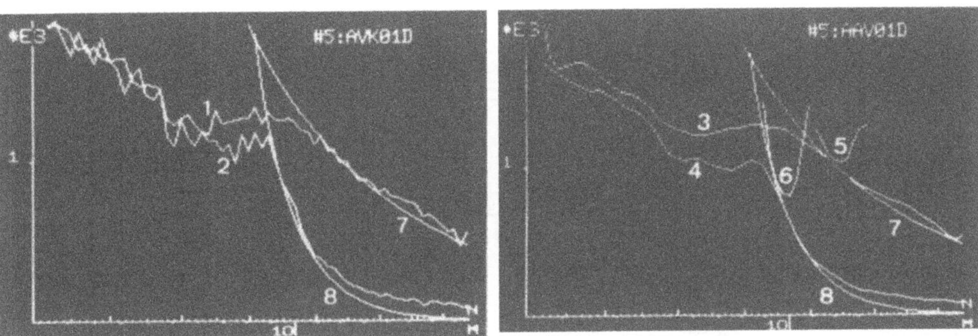

Fig. 4.27:
Two Xe-133 clearance curves (1,2) with monoexponential curve fitting (7,8) for determining the muscular blood supply in PAD. Healthy leg (2,8), diseased leg (1,7) (left). Results of interactive curve analysis with DISYA (right). For explanation of the numbered curves see text.
Sampling interval: 17 sec, counting period: 8 sec, total measurement time: 16 min

Results and Discussion

The blood supply in both legs was determined by this method in 27 patients aged between 60 and 79. With two patients the examination took place before and after unilateral sympathectomy. All cases are at angiographically determined stage III.

The blood flow rates measured for the affected extremity lie between 7 and 21 ml/100g/min with time intervals to MBF of T_m =0.6-2.1 min. The measurement values are in agreement with those in the literature dealing with diseased extremities. Ranges from 2-30 ml/100g/min with time intervals to MBF of T_m =1.1-2.3 min are given there (Fig. 4.28).

Fig. 4.28 shows the relation between time interval T_m from release of arterial occlusion to maximum washout and calculated maximum blood flow at this moment. All figures given are taken from the literature (30a,52a, 58a,99a,105a,121a,126a).

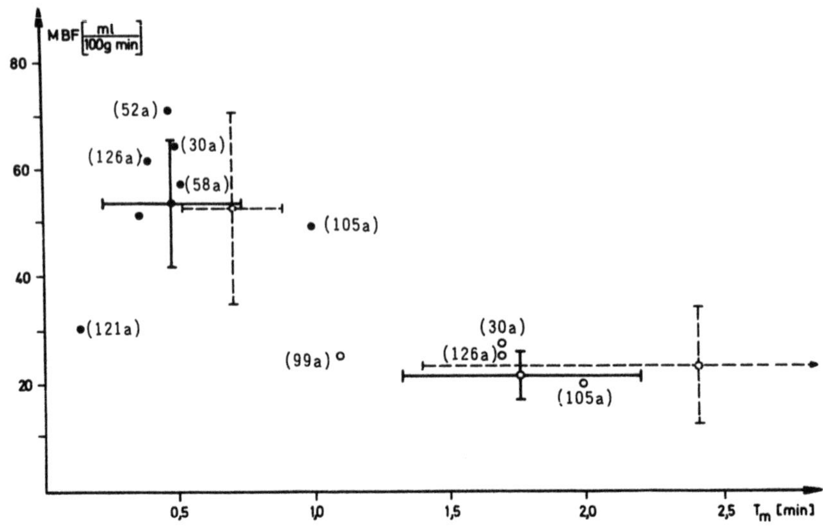

Fig. 4.28:
Maximum blood flow (MBF) and T_m in normals (•) and in peripheral arterial disease (o). Mean and S.D. (dotted: own results). Numbers refer to the literature.

In comparison, the results of our engymetric measurements with 27 patients are summarized in Fig. 4.29.

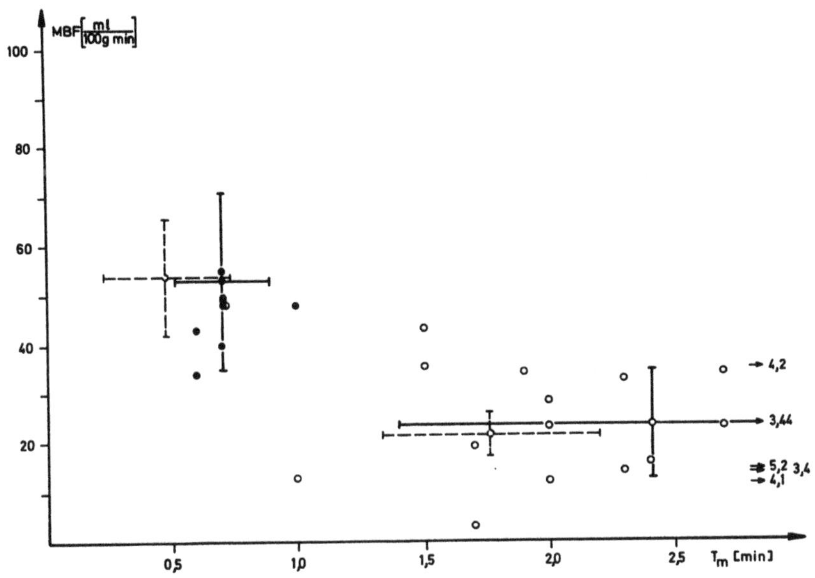

Fig. 4.29
Engymetric results for determination of normal (•) and pathological (o) MBF and T_m on 27 patients with peripheral arterial disease. Mean and S.D. (dotted: from the literature, Fig. 4.28)

Both figures 4.28,4.29 are in agreement, demonstrating the importance of T_m for the discrimination of diseased patients in addition to MBF.

For the two cases with unilateral sympathectomy there were blood supply decreases from 12 (6.5) to 10 (4) ml/100g/min on the second postoperative day. T_m was extended from 0.75 (0.6) min to 1 (0.9) min. These results are in agreement with the data by KLEMM and BECKER (109), who report on temporary worsening with subsequent improvement of the blood supply in the course of 9 months after sympathectomy.

STEINBACH et al. (190) report on further clinical applications of the Xe-133 clearance with CdTe detectors with diabetes mellitus for determining the blood supply to 4 groups of muscles (m.vastus lat., m.tib.ant., right and left) simultaneously. Using this method under stress conditions they found a reduced perfusion of the m.vastus lat. as an early indication of diabetic angiopathy.

The experience gained with MIESSY supplies functional data. These cannot be gained with angiography.

5. FURTHER APPLICATIONS

In addition to the procedures of Nuclear Medicine mentioned in the introduction, further applications of MIESSY can be expected in urology and nephrology. Determinations of side-separated clearance seem to be posible.

Obtaining the urine reflux of children would be particularly interesting. This occurs mainly with a pressure rise in the abdominal region, for instance, with micturition or defecation. Measurement values can be obtained continuously above the urethral and kidney regions by means of engymetry without disturbing the children.

Engymetric procedures are suitable for hematological examinations with radionuclides, e.g. in the determination of erythrokinetics and ferrokinetics. Thrombokinetic measurements with labeled platelets can be carried out on body regions where engymetric detectors are positioned. This also applies to the study of the kinetics of other labeled cells, such as for example white blood cells.

After the experience gained with obtaining volume changes by means of Br-82 and Tc-99m as described in Sections 4.5 - 4.7 it might be appropriate to employ engymetric examinations with developing brain edemas.

With the positioning of a number of engymetric detectors along the legs or arms the estimation of the lymph flow after appropriate labeling has been carried out successfully in preliminary studies. This procedure, especially applicable during interventions, partly follows the idea of engymetric shunt flow determination (section 4.6.1).

It seems possible to employ radionuclides in small doses emitting beta rays with the use of implanted beta detectors or ones introduced with catheters. As a result of engymetry, long integration times can be used. Continuous blood collection to determine the blood level of radioactive pharmaceuticals could be replaced by continuous observation by MIESSY.

Engymetric examinations of the kinetics of new pharmaceuticals which are radioactively labeled could be used, in particular, in tests on animals. Nuclear Medical examination procedures with MIESSY thus could be employed economically in veterinary medicine.

Extensions to radiocardiography by means of ECG triggering, as in heart blood pool scintigraphy, do not provide any great electronic difficulties. There are problems with localization. Mosaic-like groupings of individual detectors in the sense of a portable gamma camera are a possibility.

Periodic variations in the countrates have occurred in many of the long-term measurements over several days. These lead one to conclude that there are cycles. After a continuous measurement of Tl-201 kinetics over 72 hours it was easily possible to recognize the phases of falling asleep in the evening and waking up in the morning from countrate changes. It might be rewarding to employ MIESSY to examine biorhythms.

Microneurosurgical extra-intracranial bypass operations are performed as a prophylaxis for brain infarcts after transitory ischemic attacks, and after prolonged reversible attacks. Branches of the A. carotis externa anastomose by means of a small trephination with the A. cerebri media. Successful engymetric brain perfusion measurements after bolus injection of Xe-133 or Tc-99m with minidetectors over the gray matter of the hemispheres point to the possibilities of estimating intraoperatively the success of a bypass operation.

A further possible application exists in dosimetry. In contrast to dosimeters, which commonly measure integrally, the time course of the radiation exposure can be reconstructed.

Engymetry is not restricted to registering nuclear radiation fields. With adapted signal convertors it is possible to register the time courses of other physical magnitudes just as effectively.

For the future a CMOS microcomputer with low energy consumption could be integrated in the primary storage module leading to further miniaturization with increased computing power.

If particular engymetric procedures should remain clinically useful microprograms could be developed for immediate analysis of the stored signals. Final results such as clearance, glomerular filtration rate, blood supply, shunt flow etc. can be imagined to appear on a liquid crystal display like the information from modern digital multi-purpose wrist watches.

6. SUMMARY

A new, self-developed Medical Information Extraction and Storage System (MIESSY), is described. It serves to register in loco, in situ nuclear radiation fields in examinations of Nuclear Medicine. The signals thus obtained are analyzed in dialog with a personal computer system.

The programmable storage device specially developed for this purpose is battery-powered, and is carried by the patient (150,158,161). This means that continuous measurements are possible, independent of the patient's environment, and without restricting his mobility (ENGYMETRY) (158). The portable storage device is a multi-channel one. It can store measurement values from different nuclear radiation detectors simultaneously. Both short-term and long-term measurements can be carried out. This is not always possible with the usual large stationary or mobile equipment (gamma camera).

The examination methods of Nuclear Medicine are usually NON-INVASIVE. The portability of MIESSY now also permits the uncomplicated additional diagnostic employment of radioindicators during INVASIVE procedures such as operations or catheterizations. This opens up a broad field of novel applications, as, for example, intraoperative blood supply measurements of the parenchyma in the heart or brain for the immediate control of the success of bypass operations.

A new 'dialog system', DISYA, was conceived and realized for the analysis of engymetric measurement values. It favours non-algorithmic problem solving in dialog for physicians with limited knowledge of electronic data processing. It might also be of interest for experts. An extensive library of program modules for monadic and dyadic operations, graphics and data administration was developed. With a special technique it is possible to incorporate new programs in FORTRAN and PASCAL interactively into the dialog. There are possibilities for the automation of analyses. The dialog system is implemented with an inexpensive personal computer as the carrier in the sense of 'Alternative Data Processing'. The development and testing of MIESSY in clinical applications took place over a period of 6 years.

Clinical results show that engymetry can mean the extension and complementing of the usual procedures of Nuclear Medicine. In addition, MIESSY points the way to new possibilities for the employment of radioactive isotopes after HEVESY's tracer principle.

7. REFERENCES

1. Achilles, D.: Die Fouriertransformation in der Signalverarbeitung. Springer Verlag, Berlin-Heidelberg-New York, 1978.

2. Advances in imaging instrumentation. Sem. Nucl. Med. 7, No. 4: 283-365, 1977.

3. Addendum to the APPLE PASCAL Operating System Reference Manual. APPLE Computer Inc., Part 031-0100-00, 1980.

4. Addendum to the APPLE PASCAL Language Reference Manual. APPLE Computer Inc., Part 031-0101-00, 1980.

5. Ahlberg, J.H. The Theory of Splines and their Applications. Academic Press New York, 1978.

6. Akerman, M., De Tovar, G., Guiot, G.: Radioisotope cisternography and ventriculography in noncommunicating hydrocephalus. In: Cisternography and Hydrocephalus (ed. Harbert, J.C.), Charles C.Thomas, Springfield, Ill.: 483-501, 1972.

7. Albert, E., Evans, J.: Gamma ray response of a 38 mm bismuth germanate scintillator. IEEE Trans. Nucl. Sc., NS-27: 172-175, 1980.

8. Allhoff, E., Mödder, G., Engelking, R., Heising, J.: Nukliddetektorgesteuerte radikale Lymphadenektomie bei Non-Seminom-Hodentumoren. Urologie A 20: 42-45, 1981.

9. Alpert, J.S., Larsen, A.O., Lassen, N.A.: Evaluation of arterial insufficiency of the legs. A comparison of arteriography and the Xe-133 walking test. Cardiovasc. Res. 2: 161-169, 1968.

10. ANSI X3.9-1966, American National Standards Institute, Inc., New York, 1966.

11. ANSI X3.9-1978, American National Standards Institute, Inc., New York, 1978.

12. APPLE PASCAL Update APPLE Computer Inc., Part 030-0184-00, 1980.

13. APPLE II, APPLE FORTRAN Language Reference Manual. APPLE Computer Inc., Product A2D0032 (030-0118-00), 1980.

14. APPLE II, APPLE PASCAL, Operating System Reference Manual. APPLE Computer Inc., Product A2L0028 (030-0100-00), 1980.

15. APPLE II, APPLE PASCAL, Language Reference Manual. APPLE Computer Inc., Product A2L0027 (030-0101-00), 1980.

16. APPLE II Reference Manual. APPLE Computer Inc., Product A2L0001A (030-0004-01), 1979.

17. Astrup, A., Bülow, J., Madsen, J.: Skin temperature and subcutaneous adipose blood flow in man.
Scand. J. clin. Lab. Invest. 40: 135-138, 1980.

18. Bassingthwaighte, J.B.: Approaches to modeling radiocardiographic data: comments on F. Castellana's modeling of the central circulation.
In: Quantitative Nuclear Cardiography (eds. Pierson jr., R.N., Kriss, J.P. et al.)
J. Wiley & Sons, New York: 226-230, 1975.

19. Bassingthwaighte,J.B.: Physiology and theory of tracer washout techniques for the estimation of mycardial blood flow: flow estimation from tracer washout.
Progr. Cardiovasc. Dis. 20: 165-189, 1977.

20. Bassingthwaighte,J.B.: Circulatory transport and the convolution integral.
Mayo Clin. Proc. 42: 137-154, 1967.

21. Bassingthwaighte,J.B.: Plasma indicator dispersion in arteries of the human leg.
Circulation Res. 19: 332-346, 1966.

22. Bassingthwaighte,J.B.: Blood flow and diffusion through mammalian organs.
Science 167: 1347-1353, 1970.

23. Bassingthwaighte,J.B.: The measurement of blood flows and volumes by indicator dilution.
Medical Engineering (eds. Ch. D. Ray), Year Book Medical Publishers, Chicago: 246-260, 1974.

24. Bassingthwaighte,J.B.: Physiology and theory of tracer washout techniques for the estimation of mycardial blood flow: flow estimation from tracer washout.
Progr. Cardiovasc. Dis. 20: 165-189, 1977.

25. Bassingthwaighte,J.B., Ackerman,F.H., Wood,E.H.: Applications of the lagged normal density curve as a model for arterial dilution curves.
Circulation Res. 18: 398-415, 1966.

26. Bassingthwaighte,J.B., Chinard,F.P., Crone,C., Lassen,N.A., Perl,W.: Definitions, terminology for indicator dilution methods.
In: Capillary Permeability (eds. C.Crone, N.A.Lassen), Copenhagen, Ejnar Munksgaard: 665-669, 1970.

27. Bassingthwaighte,J.B., Holloway Jr.,G.A.: Estimation of blood flow with radioactive tracers.
Sem. Nucl. Med. 6: 141-161, 1976.

28. Bassingthwaighte,J.B., Knopp,T.J., Anderson,D.U.: Flow estimation by indicator dilution (bolus injection).
Circ.Res. 15: 277-290, 1970.

29. Bauer, F.L., Goos, G.: Informatik, 1. Teil.
Springer-Verlag, Berlin, Heidelberg, New York: 18, 1971.

30. Baxter, R.D.: Miniature hybrid preamplifier for CdTe detectors.
IEEE Trans. on Nucl. Science, NS-23: 493-497, 1976.

30a. Bell, G., Short, D.W.: The measurement of blood flow through muscle from the clearance of radioactive Xenon.
Surg. Gynec. Obst. 127: 61-65, 1968.

31. Berger,H.J., Davies,R.A., Batsford,W.P., Hoffer,P.B., Gottschalk,A., Zaret,B.L.: Beat-to-beat left ventricular performance assessed from the equilibrium cardiac blood pool using a computerized nuclear probe.
Circulation 63: 133-142, 1981.

32. Berman,M.: Kinetic modeling in physiology
FEBS Lett., 2, Suppl. 1, 56-57, 1969.

33. Berman,M.: The formulation and testing of models.
Ann. N. Y. Acad. Sci 108: 182-194, 1964.

34. Berman,M., Weiss,M.F.: SAAM Manual.
Washington,DC, Department of Health Education and Welfare, Publ (NIH) 78-180, 1978.

35. Bismuth Germanate.
The Harshaw Chemical Company, Crystal & Electronic Products, Solon, Ohio 44139, 1980.

36. Blahd, W.H.: History of external counting procedures.
Sem. Nucl. Med. 9: 159-163, 1979.

37. Bojsen, J., Möller, U., Christensen, P., Lippert, J.: Telemetry of radionuclide tracers by implantable thermoluminescent dosimeters on rats.
Biotelemetry II., Karger, Basel: 43-45, 1974.

38. Bojsen, J.: Biotelemetry with radionuclide tracers. In: A Handbook on Biotelemetry and Radio Tracking (eds. Amlaner jr, C.J., MacDonald, D.W.),
Pergamon Press Ltd., Oxford, 1982 (in print).

39. Bojsen, J., Vadstrup, S.: A portable external two-channel radiotelemetrical GM-detector unit, for measurements of radionuclide-tracers in vivo.
Int. J. Appl. Radiat. Isotop. 25: 161-166, 1974.

40. Bojsen, J., Vadstrup, S.: Storage telemetric system for detection of radionuclide tracers in humans.
J. Appl. Physiol. 41: 416-418, 1976.

41. Bojsen, J., Nielsen, P.E., Rasmussen, S., Parving, H.-H.: Storage telemetry of the disappearance rate of DTPA-(Sn)-Tc-99m and glomerular filtration rate by external skin surface CdTe-detectors. In: Biotelemetry IV (eds. Klewe, H.-J., Kimmich, H.P.), Döring-Druck, Braunschweig: 251-254, 1978.

42. Bojsen, J., Rossing, N.: Biotelemetry of the glomerular filtration rate (GFR) in man by external detection of DTPA -(Sn)-Tc-99m with CdTe detectors.
Nucl. Instr. Meth. 150: 49-53, 1978.

43. Boucher,Ch.A., Ahluwalia,B., Block,P.C., BrownellG.L., Beller,G.A.: Inhalation imaging with oxygen-15 labeled carbon dioxide for detection and quantification of left-to-right shunts.
Circulation 56: 632-640, 1977.

44. Bowles, K.L.: Microcomputer problem solving using PASCAL. Springer-Verlag, Berlin, Heidelberg, New York, 1977.

45. Bowles, K.L.: Beginner's guide for the UCSD PASCAL system. Byte Books, Subsidiary of McGraw-Hill, 3rd printing, Peterborough, NH03458, 1980.

46. Bracewell,R.N.: The Fourier Transform and its Applications. McGraw-Hill Book Company, New York, 1978.

47. Brauch, W.: Programmmierung mit FORTRAN. B.G. Teubner, Stuttgart, 1972.

48. Brownell,G.L., Callahan,A.B.: Transform methods for tracer data analysis. Ann. Y. A. Acad. Sci. 108: 172-181, 1964.

49. Brownell,G.L., Berman,M., Robertson,J.S.: Nomenclature for tracer kinetics. Int. J. Appl. Rad. Isotop. 19: 249-262, 1968.

50. Callahan,A.B., Pizer,S.M.: The applicability of Fourier transform analysis to biological compartmental models. In: Natural Automata and Useful Simulations (eds.: H.H.Pattee, E.A.Edelsack, L.Fein, A.B.Callahan, Spartan Books, Washington: 149-177, 1966.

51. Cerretelli, P., Blau, M., Pendergast, D., Eisenhardt, C., Rennie, D.W.: Cadmium telluride Xe-133 clearance detector for muscle blood flow studies. IEEE Trans. Nucl. Sci., NS-25: 620-623, 1978.

52. Chen, Chi-tsong: One-dimensional digital signal processing. Marcel Dekker, Inc., New York, Basel, 1979.

52a. Christensen, N.J.: The significance of work load and injected volume in Xenon 133 measurement of muscular blood flow. Acta Med. Scand. 183: 445-447, 1968.

53. Cobelli,C., Romanin-Jacur,G.: Controllability, observability and structural identifiability of multi input and multi output biological compartmental systems. IEEE Transactions on Biomedical Engineering, Vol. BME-23. no.2: 93-100, 1976.

54. Coulam,C.M., Warner,H.R., Wood,E.H., Bassirgthwaighte,J.B.: A transfer function analysis of coronary and renal circulation calculated from upstream and downstream indicator-dilution curves. Circ. Res. 19: 879-890, 1966.

55. Davidson, H.G., Gudbjerg, C.E., Thomsen, G.: Complications of selective angiocardiography and percutaneous transarterial aortography. Acta chir. scand.: 283, Suppl., 168-181, 1961.

56. Davis,G.C., Paulsen,A.W., Frederickson,E.L.: The effect of total peripheral resistance on the parameters of the lagged normal model of indicator-dilution curves. Comp. Biomed. Res. 10: 323-331, 1977.

57. De Blanc jr., H.J., Natarajan, T.K., James, A.E., Wagner jr., H.N.: Computer-assisted quantitative cisternography and ventriculography.
In: Cisternography and Hydrocephalus (ed. Harbert, J.C.), Charles C. Thomas, Springfield-Ill.: 471-482, 1972.

58. Denert, E., Hesse, W.: Projektmodell und Projektbibliothek: Grundlagen zuverlässiger Software-Entwicklung und Dokumentation.
Informatik-Spektrum 3: 215-228, 1980.

58a. DeRoo, M., Bossaert, A., Amery, A., Verstraete, M.: Preliminary results of the Xe-133 exploration of the arterial vascularization of the legs.
J. Belge Radiol. 52: 52-58, 1969.

59. Echtermeyer, V., Brenneisen, W., Pretschner, D.P., Kolbow, H.: Eine neue Methode zur Diagnostik des Compartment-Syndroms.
Chir. Forum '81 f. exp. u. klin. Forschung, Langenbecks Archiv f. Chirurgie, Suppl.: 121-125, 1981.

60. Echtermeyer, V., Godt, P., Muhr, G.: Das posttraumatische Muskel-Kompressionssyndrom, Pathophysiologie und Technik der Dekompression.
Hefte Unfallheilk. 148: 492-497, 1980.

61. Emde, H., Huber, G., Piepgras, U.: Der Stellenwert der Liquorraum-Szintigraphie im Vergleich zur kranialen Computertomographie.
Der Nuklearmediziner 3: 152-170, 1979.

62. Endres, A.: Methoden der Programm- und Systemkonstruktion.
Informatik-Spektrum 3: 156-171, 1980.

63. Enger, E.: Programmieren mit PASCAL. 1.-5. Teil.
Elektronik 29, Heft 4, 5, 6, 7, 8, 1980.

64. Entzian, W., Palma, A., Kolberg, T.: Bedeutung der szintigraphischen Untersuchung der Liquordynamik für neurochirurgische Patienten.
Der Nuklearmediziner 1: 107-116, 1978.

65. Essig, H.: Benutzerfreundlichkeit/Benutzerakzeptanz. Zur Situation eines interdisziplinären Forschungsgebietes.
Universität Hamburg, Fachbereich Informatik IFI-HH-B-65/79, 1979.

66. Essig, H.: Benutzerfreundlichkeit.
Informatik-Spektrum 4: 51-52, 1981.

67. Evert,C.F., Randall,M.J.: Formulation and computation of compartment models.
J. Pharm. Sci. 59: 403-409, 1970.

68. Ewins, J.H. Friedland, S.S.: Solid state detectors in behavioral studies.
IEEE Trans. Nucl. Science, NS-17: 275-281, 1970.

69. Feinendegen,L.E.: Minimal transit times.
Nucl.-Med. XVII: 185-193, 1978.

70. Fischer, H.: Pathophysiologie und Therapie des venösen Stauungsödems.
Therapiewoche 28: 857-875, 1978.

71. Frick, M., Rösler, H., Mumenthaler, M., Steinziepa, K.: Der prognostische Wert des Radiocisternogrammes für die Shuntoperation bei Hydrocephalus communicans internus.
Fortschr. a. d. Geb. der Röntgenstr. 121: 634-643, 1974.

72. Friedland, S.S., Benary, V., Ewins, J.H., Katzenstein, H.S.: In vivo silicon detectors, in vivo preamplifiers and their applications.
IEEE Trans. Nucl. Sci., NS-19: 244-251, 1972.

73. Föllinger, O.: Regelungstechnik, Einführung in die Methoden und ihre Anwendung.
Elitera-Verlag, Berlin, 1972.

74. Friedman, B.H., Siegel, M.E., Rhodes, B.A., Wagner jr., H.N.: Venous haemodynamics.
In: Dynamic Studies with Radioisotopes in Medicine 1974, IAEA, Vienna: 105-112, 1975.

75. Fuhrmeister, U.: Spinaler Infusionstest und verwandte Methoden lumbaler Druckmessung.
In: Cerebrospinalflüssigkeit - CSF (Hrsg. Dommasch, D., Mertens, H.G.),
Georg Thieme-Verlag, Stuttgart-New York: 242-253, 1980.

76. Garcia, D.A., Entine, G., Tow, D.E.: Detection of small bone abscesses with a high-resolution cadmium telluride probe.
J. Nucl. Med. 15: 892-895, 1974.

77. Gates,G.F., Orme,H.W., Dore,E.K.: Cardiac shunt assessment in children with macroaggregated albumin technetium-99m.
Radiology 112: 649-653, 1974.

78. Gates,G.F., Orme,H.W., Dore,E.K.: Measurement of cardiac shunting with technetium-labeled albumin aggregates.
J. Nucl. Med. 12: 746-749, 1971.

79. Gesellschaft für Nuklearmedizin - Europa- : 19th Int. Ann. Meeting, Precongress Teaching Courses: Data Processing in Nuclear Medicine, Bern, 31.8.-4.9. 1981.

80. Geyer, J.: 32-Bit-Microcomputer besitzt neuartige Architektur.
Elektronik 5: 59-66, 1981.

81. Goodwin, D.A., Bushberg, J.T., Doherty, P.W., Lipton, M.J., Conley, F.K., Diamanti, C.I., Meares, C.F.: Indium-111-labeled autologous platelets for location of vascular thrombi in humans.
J. Nucl. Med. 19: 626-634, 1978.

82. Gudbjerg, C.E., Christensen, J.: Dissection of aortic wall in retrograde lumbar aortography.
Acta radiol. 55, 364-368, 1961.

83. Guller,B., Yipintsoi,T., Orvis,A.L., Bassingthwaighte, J.B.: Myocardial sodium extraction at varied coronary flows in the dog
Circ. Res. 37: 359-378, 1975.

84. Gurewich, V.: Pathogenesis of thromboembolism. In: Postoperative Thromboembolie-Prophylaxe (Hrsg. Papst, H.W., Maurer, G.),
F.K. Schattauer-Verlag, Stuttgart, New York: 31-37, 1977.

85. Hackstein, H.: Programmieren mit Objekten. Elektronik 11: 71-74, 1981.

86. Hartmann, F.: Konjekturen und Indikationen als Formen ärztlichen Urteils, Vorbereitung eines kritischen Empirismus in der Medizin. 3. Arbeitsgespräch des Arbeitskreises für Methodologie der klinischen Medizin, Stuttgart, 1981. Archiv für Medizinforschung, Bd. IV, Burgverlag, Tecklenburg (im Druck).

87. Harris,Th.R., Newman,E.V.: An analysis of mathematical models of circulatory indicator-dilution curves. J. Appl. Physiol. 28: 840-850, 1970.

88. Harrison,K.S., Liu,X., Han,S.-T., Camargo,E.E., Wagner,Jr.,H.N.: Evaluation of a miniature CdTe detector for monitoring left ventricular function. Eur. J. Nucl. Med. 7: 204-206, 1982.

89. Hassan, M.A.: A semiconductor radiation pill. In: Biotelemetry IV (eds. Klewe, H.-J., Kimmich, H.P.), Döring-Druck, Braunschweig: 61-64, 1978.

90. Hassan, M.A., Pearce, G., Edwards, J.P.N.: A radiotelemetry pill for the measurement of ionising radiation using a mercuric iodide detector. Phys. Med. Biol. 23: 302-308, 1978.

91. Henninges, D., Friedel, B., Müller, D., Zeitler, E.: Die 133-Xenonmuskelclearance im Vergleich mit Belastungsoszillographie, Ultraschalldopplertechnik und Venenverschluss- plethysmographie. In: Diagnostik mit Isotopen bei arteriellen und venösen Durchblutungsstörungen der Extremitäten (Hrsg. Zeitler, E.), Verlag Hans Huber, Bern, Stuttgart, Wien: 88-95, 1973.

92. Höhne, K.H., Pfeiffer, G.: The role of the physician - computer interaction in the acquisition and interpretation of scintigraphic data. Meth. Inform. Med. 13: 65-70, 1974.

93. Hoffer, P.B., Berger, H.J., Steidley, J., Brendel, A.F., Gottschalk, A., Zaret, B.L.: A miniature cadmium telluride detector module for continuous monitoring of left-ventricular function. Radiology 138: 477-481, 1981.

94. Horst, W.: Klinische Radiojoddiagnostik der Schilddrüsenerkrankungen. In: Strahlenbiologie, Strahlentherapie, Nuklearmedizin und Krebsforschung, Ergebnisse 1952-1958 (Hrsg. Schinz, H.R.), Georg Thieme Verlag, Stuttgart: 789-940, 1959.

95. Hundeshagen, H.: Radiokardiographie. Dr. A. Hüthig Verlag, Heidelberg 1970.

96. Jacquez, J.A.: Compartmental analysis in biology and medicine. Elsevier Publ. Co., Amsterdam, London, New York, 1972.

97. Jensen, K., Wirth, H.: PASCAL user manual and report. Second corrected reprint of the 2nd edition, Springer-Verlag, New York, Heidelberg, Berlin, 1978.

98. Jordan, W., Urban, H.: Strukturierte Programmierung. Springer-Verlag, Berlin, Heidelberg, New York, 1978.

99. Jordan, K.: Grundlagen der Strahlenmesstechnik. In: Handbuch der med. Radiologie, Bd. 15, Teil 1A (Hrsg. Hundeshagen, H.), Springer-Verlag, Berlin, Heidelberg: 131-206, 1980.

99a. Kampik, E.: Möglichkeiten und Grenzen bei der Differenzierung arterieller Obliterationen mit der Xenonclearance. In: Diagnostik mit Isotopen bei arteriellen und venösen Durchblutungsstörungen der Extremitäten, (ed. E. Zeitler), Verlag H.Huber, Bern: 54-60, 1973.

100. Karlsberg,R.P., Gelezunas,V.L., Lyons,K.P.: Highly localized in vivo measurement of myocardial perfusion with avalanche radiation detectors. Circulation 65: 54-61, 1982.

101. Katzan, H. jr.: APL user's guide. Van Nostrand Reinhold Co., New York, 1971.

102. Katzan, H. jr.: FORTRAN 77. Van Nostrand Reinhold Co., New York, 1978.

103. Kakkar, V.V., Nicolaides, A.N., Renney, J.T.G., Friend, J.R., Clarke, M.B.: I-125 labeled fibrinogen test adapted for routine screening for deep-vein thrombosis. Lancet 1: 540-542, 1970.

104. Kakkar, V.V.: Diagnosis of deep vein thrombosis. In: Postop. Thromboembolie-Prophylaxe, (Hrsg. Pabst, H.W., Maurer, G.), F.K. Schattauer-Verlag, Stuttgart, New York: 39-47, 1977.

105. Kendall,M.G.: Time Series. Griffin, London, 1973.

105a. Kirsch, G., Höwner, B.: Xenon 133 Muskelclearance bei peripheren arteriellen Durchblutungsstörungen. Radiobiol. Radiother. 2: 215-224, 1977.

106. Klee,H.: Einsatz eines Mikrocomputers in der Nuklearmedizin zur interaktiven Analyse engymetrischer Zeit-Aktivitäts-Histogramme. Universität Heidelberg - Fachhochschule Heilbronn, Studiengang Medizinische Informatik, Diplomarbeit, 1982.

107. Kety, S.S.: Measurement of regional circulation by local clearance of radioactive sodium. Amer. Heart J. 38: 321-328, 1949.

108. Kiessling, D.R., Pretschner, D.P., Hundeshagen, H.: Zur Bestimmung der Auswurffraktion mit der Einzelsondenmesstechnik im Vergleich zu Angiokardiographie und Herzbinnenraum-Szintigraphie. In: Nuklearmedizin, Computer Assisted Functional Analysis (Hrsg. Schmidt, H.A.E., Rösler, H.), F.K. Schattauer-Verlag, Stuttgart-New York: 413-416, 1982.

109. Klemm, J., Becker, H.M.: Die Beurteilung chirurgischer Behandlungsergebnisse bei arteriellen Durchblutungsstörungen mit der 133-Xenon-Muskelclearance. In: Diagnostik mit Isotopen bei arteriellen und venösen Durchblutungsstörungen der Extremitäten, (Hrsg. Zeitler, E.), Verlag Hans Huber, Bern, Stuttgart, Wien: 69-73, 1973.

110. Knopp,T.J., Bassingthwaighte,J.B.: Effect of flow on transpulmonary circulatory transport functions.
J. Appl. Physiol. 27: 36-43, 1969.

111. Knötgen, H.G., Füger, G.F., Gell, G.: Intraventricular I-131-hippurate in hydrocephalus.
In: Cisternography and Hydrocephalus (ed. Harbert, J.C.), Charles C. Thomas, Springfield-Ill.: 521-544, 1972.

112. Kolendorf, K., Bojsen, J., Jorgensen, K.: Storage telemetry of subcutaneous absorption of 125-I-NPH-insulin. In: Biotelemetry IV (Hrsg. Klewe, H.-J., Kimmich, H.P.),
Döring-Druck, Druckerei u. Verlag, Braunschweig: 239-242, 1980.

113. Koch, G.R.: Systematisches Softwareengineering für Microcomputer, 1.-2. Teil.
Elektronik 28, Heft 21: 49-56, Heft 22: 72-78, 1979.

114. Koffmann, E.B.: Problem solving and structured programming in PASCAL.
Addison-Wesley Publishing Co., Reading, Mass., 1981.

115. Korvald, E., Abildgaard, U., Fagerhol, M.K.: Major operations, hemostatic parameters and venous thrombosis.
Thromb. Res. 4: 147-154, 1974.

116. Kuikka,J., Lehtovirta,P., Kuikka,E., Rekonen,A.: Application of the modified gamma function to the calculation of cardiopulmonary blood pools in radiocardiography.
Phys. Med. Biol. 19: 692-700, 1974.

117. Kupka, I., Wilsing, N.: Dialogsprachen.
B.G. Teubner, Stuttgart, 1975.

118. Lanz, U.: Ischämische Muskelnekrosen.
Hefte Unfallheilk. 139:C 1-70, 1979.

119. Larson, O.A.: Xe-133 methods for determining peripheral blood flow and blood pressure in patients with occlusive arterial disease.
Angiology 23: 153-162, 1972.

120. Lassen, N.A., Hoedt-Rasmussen, K., Lindbjerg, I., Pedersen, F., Munck, D.: Muscle blood flow determined by use of Xe-133.
Scand. J. Clin. lab. Invest. 15, Suppl. 76: 61, 1963.

121. Lassen, N.A., Lindbjerg, I.F., Dahn, I.: Validity of the Xe-133-method for measurement of muscle blood flow evaluated by simultaneous venous occlusion plethysmography: observations in the calf of normal man and in patients with occlusive vascular disease.
Circ. Res. 16: 287-293, 1965.

121a. Lassen, N.A., Lindbjerg, J., Munk, O.: Measurement of blood flow through skeletal muscle by intramuscular injection of Xenon-133.
Lancet 1: 686-694, 1968.

122. Lassen, N.A., Perl, W.: Tracer kinetic methods in medical physiology.
Raven Press, New York, 1979.

123. Laurent,J.P., Lawner,P., Simeone,F.A., Fink,E.: Pentobarbital changes compartmental contribution to cerebral blood flow. J. Neurosurg. 56: 504-510, 1982.

124. Leth, A., Binder, C.: The distribution volume of Br-82 as a measurement of the extracellular fluid volume in normal persons. Scand. J. clin. Lab. Invest. 25: 291-297, 1970.

125. Lewis, T.G.: PASCAL programming for the APPLE. Reston Publishing Co., Inc., Reston, Virginia, 1981.

126. Lichtlen, P.R.: Langzeitresultate der Bypass-Chirurgie. In: Koronarangiographie (Hrsg. Lichtlen, P.R.), Perimed Verlag Dr. med. D. Straube, Erlangen: 448-463, 1979.

126a. Lindbjerg, J.F.: Diagnostic application of the 133-Xenon method in peripheral arterial disease. Scand. J. Clin. Lab. Invest. 17: 589-599, 1965.

127. Lying-Turell, U., Söderborg, B.: Quantitative methods of estimating CSF flow. In: Cisternography and Hydrocephalus. (ed.: Harbert, J.C.), Charles C. Thomas, Springfield, Ill: 503-511, 1972.

128. Malone, J.M., Leal, J.M., Moore, W.S., Henry, R.E., Daly, M.J., Patton, D.D., Childers, S.J.: The 'gold standard' for amputation level selection: Xenon-133 clearance. J. Surg. Res. 30: 449-455, 1981.

129. Martini, M.: Semiconductor radiation probes for nuclear medicine and radiobiology, the state of the art. IEEE Trans. Nucl. Sci., NS-20: 294-309, 1972.

130. Matsen III, F.A.: Compartmental syndromes. Grune & Stratton, New York, London, Toronto, Sydney, San Francisco, 1980.

131. Matsen III, F.A., Winquist, R.A., Krugmire jr, R.B.: Diagnosis and management of compartmental syndromes. J. Bone Joint Surg. 59-A: 286-291, 1980.

132. McAfee, J.G.: A survey of complications of abdominal aortography. Radiology 68: 825-838, 1957.

133. McLeod,J., Osborn,J.: Physiological simulation in general- and in particular. In: Natural Automata and Useful Simulations, (eds.: H.H.Pattee, E.A.Edelsack, L.Fein, A.B.Callahan), Spartan Books, Washington: 127-138, 1966.

134. Mostbeck, A., Partsch, H., Peschl, L.: Änderungen der Blutvolumenverteilung im Ganzkörper unter physikalischen und pharmakologischen Massnahmen. VASA 6: 137-142, 1977.

135. Mubarak, S.J., Owen, C.A., Hargens, A.R., Garetto, L.P., Akeson, W.H.: Acute compartment syndromes: Diagnosis and treatment with the aid of the wick catheter. J. Bone Joint Surg. 60-A: 1091-1095, 1978.

136. Müller-Brand, J., Friedrich, R., Duckert, F., Gruber, U.F., Schmitt, H.E.:
Tendenzen in der nuklearmedizinischen Thrombosediagnostik.
Schweiz. med. Wschr. 106: 78-81, 1976.

137. Nickles,R.J., Nelson,P.J., Polcyn,R.E., Holden,J.E., Kiuru,A.J.:
Radioactive gases in the evaluation of left ventricular function.
In: Nuclear Cardiology: Principles and Methods (eds.: A.N.Serafini, A.J.Gilson,W.M.Smoak), Plenum Medical Book Company, New York, London: 217-230, 1977.

138. Otto, H., Göbel, S., Bock, W.J., Strötges, M.W.: Funktionskontrollen ventrikulo-atrialer und ventrikulo-peritonealer Anastomosen mit Tc-99-Albumin.
Nuklearmediziner 2: 103-106, 1978.

139. Palma, A., Kolberg, T.: Neue Aspekte der Liquordynamik beim Menschen durch sequentielle Kameraszintigraphie und Auswertung mit Digitalanalysator, Teil I: Methodik und physiologische Verhältnisse.
Acta Neurochir. 36: 9-28, 1977.

140. Papoulis,A.: Signal Analysis.
McGraw-Hill Book Company, New York, 1977.

141. Partain, C.L. Staab, E.V., Wu, M.P., Alderson, P.O., Rujanavech, N., Siegel, B.A.: Cerebrospinal fluid kinetics in normal human volunteers via radionuclide imaging and mathematical modelling.
In: Medical Radionuclide Imaging. Vol. II,
IAEA, Vienna: 371-378, 1977.

142. Pavel, D.G., Zimmer, M. et al.: In vivo labeling of red blood cells with Tc-99m: a new approach to blood pool visualization.
J. Nucl. Med. 18: 305-308, 1977.

143. Pertynski, T., Radecki, W., Bialobrzeski, J.: Oviduct patency control by means of Xe-133-solution
Nucl. Med. XV: 46-49, 1976.

144. Pfeiffer, G.: Entwurf und Implementierung eines Dialogsystems zur Erzeugung interaktiver Bildverarbeitungssysteme in der Medizin.
Dissertation, Fachbereich Informatik, Universität Hamburg, 1981.

145. Pfeiffer, G., Höhne, K.H.: Improvements of programming efficiency in medical image processing by a dialog language.
Proc. of MIE 78, Lecture Notes in Medical Informatics, Springer-Verlag, New York: 221-231, 1978.

146. Pfeiffer, G., Höhne, K.H.: A dialog language for interactive processing of scintigraphic data.
In: Proc. IVth Int. Conf. on Inf. Proc. in Scintigraphy (eds. Raynaud, C., Todd-Pokropek, A.E.), Orsay: 221-231, 1975.

147. Pfeiffer,G.: Erzeugung interaktiver Bildverarbeitungssysteme im Dialog.
Informatik-Fachberichte (ed.: W.Bauer), Vol.51, Springer Verlag, Berlin, Heidelberg, New York, 1982.

148. Piepsz, A., Ham, H.R., Hall, M., Frondeville, J.L., Ectors, M.: GFR measurement in children by means of a CdTe portable detector.
J. Nucl. Med. 22: P 37, 1981.

149. Pretschner, D.P., Bornemann, H., Reuter, Th.D., Jordan, K.: Einsatz eines Minidetektors zur Diagnostik bei Thrombosierungen und kongenitalen Herzvitien. In: Der klin. Wert der Methoden der Nuklearmedizin, (abstract), 16th Ann. Meeting Soc. Nucl. Med., Madrid: 152, 1978.

150. Pretschner, D.P., Gettner, U.: Eine neue Vorrichtung zur kontinuierlichen Erfassung orts- und zeitabhängiger Aktivitätsverteilungen im Menschen. In: Nuklearmedizin, Nuklearmedizin und Biokybernetik, (Hrsg. Öff, K., Schmidt, H.A.E.), Bd. 2, Verhandlungsber. 14. Int. Jahrestag. Ges. f. Nucl.med., Berlin, 15.-18. Sept. 1976, Medico-Informationsdienste, Berlin: 502-505, 1978.

151. Pretschner, D.P., Hundeshagen, H., Kallfelz, H.C., Freymann, R.: Zur radiokardiographischen Bestimmung von Links-Rechts-Shunts. In: Nuklearmedizin, Nuklearmedizin und Biokybernetik, (Hrsg. Öff, K., Schmidt, J.A.E.), Bd. I, Medico-Informationsdienste, Berlin: 460-464, 1978.

152. Pretschner, D.P.: FORTRAN - Pflicht für Nuklearmediziner? In: Nuklearmedizin, Stand und Zukunft (Hrsg. Schmidt, H.A.E., Woldring, M.), F.K. Schattauer-Verlag, Stuttgart-New York: 827- 831, 1978.

153. Pretschner, D.P., Freihorst, J., Gleitz, C.D., Hundeshagen, H.: 201-Tl myocardial scintigraphy: a 3-dimensional model for the improved quantification of zones with decreased uptake. In: Inf. Proc.in Med. Imaging (eds. Di Paola, R., Kahn, E.), INSERM, Vol. 88: 409-426, 1979.

154. Pretschner, D.P., Freihorst, J., Gleitz, C.-D., Hundeshagen, H.: A computer generated 3-D model of the left ventricle for quantification of myocardial morphology and function using radiopharmaceuticals. In: Computers in Cardiology (eds. Ripley, K.L., Ostrow, H.G.), IEEE, Genf: 415-418, 1979.

155. Pretschner, D.P.: Nuclear medicine in Europe, considerations of present status and future trends. Eur. J. Nucl. Med. 5: 175-184, 1980.

156. Pretschner, D.P., Gettner, U., Brenneisen, W., Jordan, K., Hundeshagen, H.: Nuklearmedizinische Engymetrie zur Bestimmung von Änderungen des Extrazellulärraumes der unteren Extremitäten. In: Nuklearmedizin, Nuklearmedizin im interdisziplinären Bezug (Hrsg.: Schmidt, H.A.E., Wolf, F., Mahlstedt, J.), F.K. Schattauer-Verlag, Stuttgart-New York: 303-306, 1981.

157. Pretschner, D.P.: Planar imaging and picture analysis in nuclear medicine. In: Digital Image Processing in Medicine (ed. Höhne, K.H.), Springer-Verlag, Berlin, Heidelberg, New York: 149-195, 1981.

158. Pretschner, D.P.: Ein neues System zur Erfassung und Auswertung von Kernstrahlungsfeldern bei nuklearmedizinischen Untersuchungen (Engymetrie). In: Systeme und Signalverarbeitung in der Nuklearmedizin (Hrsg. Pöppl, S.J., Pretschner, D.P.), Springer-Verlag, Berlin, Heidelberg, New York: 74-95, 1981.

159. Pretschner, D.P., Pfeiffer, G.: Erzeugung einer Kommandosprache für nuklearmedizinische Signal- und Bildverarbeitung aus einem allgemeinen Dialogsystem.
In: Systeme und Signalverarbeitung in der Nuklearmedizin (Hrsg. Pöppl, S.J., Pretschner, D.P.), Springer-Verlag, Berlin, Heidelberg, New York: 187-204, 1981.

160. Pretschner, D.P.: Prinzipien parametrischer Darstellung der Herzfunktion in der Nuklearmedizin.
Der Nuklearmediziner 3: 91-106, 1980.

161. Pretschner, D.P.: Vorrichtung zur Bestimmung der Strahlung einer radioaktiv markierten, in den menschlichen Körper eingebrachten Substanz mit einem Detektor und einer einen digitalen Speicher enthaltenden Auswerteschaltung
Deutsches Patent Nr. 2641039, 1976.

162. Pretschner, D.P., Gettner, U., Klee, J.: Engymetric biosignal analysis in Nuclear Medicine.
World Congress on Medical Physics and Biomedical Engineering, Hamburg, 1982 (in press).

163. Puschert, W., Scholz, H. M.: Y-ray spectra detected with HgI_2 at room temperature.
Appl. Phys. Lett. 28: 357-359, 1976.

164. Reichertz, P.L.: Auswirkungen der elektronischen Datenverarbeitung auf die Struktur der Medizin.
Arzneim. Forsch. 21: 173-181, 1971.

165. Reichertz, P.L.: Medizinische Informatik, Aufgaben, Wege und Bedeutung.
IBM Newsletter 23, Heft 215: 567-576, 1973.

166. Reichertz, P.L. : Sinn und Kriterien einer zeitgerechten Datenverarbeitung im Dialog.
In: Interaktive Datenverarbeitung in der Medizin (Hrsg. Wagner, G., Köhler, C.O.),
F.K. Schattauer Verlag, Stuttgart: 21-39, 1976.

166a. Reichertz, P.L.: The challenge of medical informatics: delusions or new perspectives.
Med. Inform. 7: 57-66, 1982.

166b. Reichertz, P.L.: Future developments of data processing in health care.
Meth. Inform. Med. 21: 55-58, 1982.

167. Reinsch, C.H.: Smoothing by spline functions.
Num. Mathem. 10: 177-183, 1967.

168. Rhodes, B.A.: Radiopharmaceuticals.
In: Cardiovascular Nuclear Medicine (Eds.: H.W. Strauss, B. Pitt), 2nd ed., The C.V. Mosby Company, St.Louis-Toronto-London: 57-75, 1979.

169. Rollo, F.D. (ed.): Nuclear Medicine Physics, Instrumentations, and Agents.
The C.V. Mosby Company, Saint-Louis, 1977.

170. Rosen,L., Silverman,N.R.: Videodensitometric measurements of blood flow using coss-correlation techniques.
Radiology 109: 305-310, 1973.

171. Rossing, N., Bojsen, J., Frederiksen, P.L.: The glomerular filtration rate determined with Tc-99m-DTPA and a portable cadmium telluride detector.
Scand. J. Clin. Lab. Invest. 38: 23-28, 1978.

172. Sampson, W.F.D., Macleod, M.A., Warren, D.: External monitoring of kidney transplant function using Tc-99m(Sn)DTPA.
J. Nucl. Med. 22: 411-416, 1981.

173. Sanders, T.P., Sanders, T.D., Gallagher, E.J.: Quantitative studies of CSF dynamics. In: Cisternography and Hydrocephalus (ed. Harbert, J.C.),
Charles C. Thomas, Publ., Springfield, Ill.: 463-470, 1972.

174. Schieber, M.: Fabrication of HgI_2 nuclear detectors.
Nucl. Instr. Meth. 144: 469-477, 1977.

175. Schneider, W., Fischer, H.: Die chronisch-venöse Insuffizienz.
4. Auflage, Enke-Verlag, Stuttgart, 1969.

175a. Schöner, W.F., Pretschner, D.P., Dietz, H., Hundeshagen, H.: Engymetrische Erfassung der Liquorkinetik bei Hydrocephalus communicans und occlusus vor und nach der Implantation von Ventrikel-drainierenden Systemen.
In: Nuklearmedizin, Computer Assisted Functional Analysis (eds. H.A.E. Schmidt, H. Rössler), F.K.Schattauer Verlag, Stuttgart-New York: 593-597, 1982.

176. Schörner, W., Schartl, M., Felix, R.: Funktionsszintigraphische Untersuchung zur Beurteilung der Umverteilung regionaler Blutvolumina durch Nitroglycerin.
Z. Kardiol., 1982 (in press).

177. Schossberger, P.F., Touya, J.J.: Dynamic cisternography in normal dogs and in human beings.
Neurology 26: 254-260, 1976.

178. Scholz, H.: On crystallization by temperature-gradient reversal.
Acta Electron. 17: 69-73, 1974.

179. Schuchmann, H.-R.: Personal Computing als alternative Datenverarbeitung.
Elektron. Rechenanl. 23: 51-60, 1981.

180. Schulte, M.: Erkrankung der Arterien. In: Lehrbuch der Inneren Medizin (Hrsg. Gross, R., Schölmerich, P.), 5.Aufl.
F.K. Schattauer Verlag, Stuttgart, New York: 399-406, 1977.

181. Seelmann-Eggebert, W., Pfennig, G., Münzel, H.: Nuklidkarte.
Kernforschungszentrum Karlsruhe, 4. Aufl., 1974.

182. Shah, A.: Storage Telemetry: Session Introduction.
Biotelemetry II.,
Karger, Basel: 62-63, 1974.

183. Shipley, R.A., Clark, R.E.: Tracer methods for in vivo kinetics.
Academic Press, New York, London, 1972.

184. Siegel, M.E., Wagner jr., H.N.: Radioactive tracers in peripheral vascular disease.
Sem. Nucl. Med. VI: 253-278, 1976.

185. Siffert, P.: Current possibilities and limitations of cadmium telluride detectors.
Nucl. Instr. Meth. 150: 1-12, 1978.

186. Smith, R.S., Sampson, W.F.D., Warren, D.J.: Evaluation of miniaturised cadmium telluride detectors in renal transplant renography.
Nucl. Med. Commun. 2: 21-25, 1981.

187. Smith, R.S., Sampson, W.F.D., Lee, H.A., Slapak, M., Warren, D.J.: Continuous monitoring of renal transplant function by external forearm counting.
Transplant. Proc. XIII: 668-673, 1981.

188. Sorenson,J.A., Phelps,M.E.: Physics in Nuclear Medicine.
Grune & Stratton, New York, 1980.

189. Steele,P., Kirch,D., Vogel,R.: Evaluation of central circulatory dynamics with the radionuclide angiocardiogram.
In: Cardiovascular Nuclear Medicine (eds.: H.W.Strauss, B.Pitt), 2nd ed., The C.V.Mosby Company, St. Louis-Toronto-London: 105-125, 1979.

190. Steinbach, J.J., Pendergast, D., Blau, M.: Muscle blood flow in insulin dependent patients with diabetes mellitus using small solid state CdTe detectors and Xenon-133.
J. Nucl. Med. 22: P 48, 1981.

191. Strashun, A., Horowitz, S.F., Goldsmith, S.J., Teichholz, L.E., Dicker, A., Miceli, K., Gorlin, R.: Noninvasive detection of left ventricular dysfunction with a portable electrocardiographic gated scintillation probe device.
Amer. J. Cardiol. 47: 610-617, 1981.

192. Strauss,H.W., Hurley,P.J., Rhodes,B.A., Wagner Jr.,H.N.: Quantification of right-to-left transpulmonary shunts in man.
J. Lab. & Clin. Med. 74: 597-607, 1969.

193. System/360 Continuous System Modeling Program, User's Manual, Program Number 360a-Cx-16X, GH20-0367-4, I.B.M. 1972.

194. Tamer,D.M., Watson,D.D., Kenny,P.J., Janowitz,W.R., Gelband,H., Gilson,A.J.: Noninvasive detection and quantification of left-to-right shunts in children using oxygen-15 labeled carbon dioxide.
Circulation 56: 626-631, 1977.

195. Tenenbaum, A.M., Augenstein, M.J.: Data structures using PASCAL.
Prentice-Hall, Inc., Englewood Cliffs, N.J. 07632, 1981.

196. Todd-Pokropek, A.E., Plummer, D., Pizer, S.M.: Modularity and command languages in medical computing.
In: Information Processing in Med. Imaging (eds. Brill, A.B., Price, R.R., McClain, W.J., Larday, M.W.),
ORNL/BCTIC-2: 426-455, 1978.

197. Tscherne, H., Westermann, K., Trentz, O., Pretschner, D.P., Mellmann, J.: Thromboembolische Komplikationen und ihre Prophylaxe beim Hüftgelenkersatz.
Unfallheilkunde 81: 178-187, 1978.

198. Vincoff, M.N.: Radiation Resistance of the COS/MOS CD 4000 A Series.
RCA, Digital Integrated Circuits, Appl. Note, ICAN-6224, 1974.

199. Vogel, S., Synowitz, H.-J., Lommatzsch, P., Thierfelder, Ch., Correns, H.-J., Seidel, G., Bartho, H., Matauschek, K., Scherd, K.: Die klinische Anwendung von Halbleiterdetektorsonden - neue Möglichkeiten nuklearmedizinischer Diagnostik.
Dt. Gesundh.-Wesen 34: 1886-1892, 1979.

200. Wagner Jr.,H.H.: Use of the nuclear stethoscope to monitor ventricular function.
Practical Cardiology 7: 113-129, 1981.

201. Wagner, H.N., Rigo, P., Baxter, R.H., Alderson, P.O., Douglass, K.H., Householder, D.F.: Monitoring ventricular function at rest and during exercise with a nonimaging detector.
Amer. J. Cardiol. 43: 975-979, 1979.

202. Walder, D.N.: A technique for investigating the blood supply of muscle during exercise.
Brit. Med. J. I: 255-258, 1958.

203. Walford, G.V., Parker, R.P.: The development and application of coaxical CdTe medical probes for use in the clinical environment.
IEEE Trans. Nucl. Science, NS-20: 318-328, 1972.

204. Watson, D.D.: Shunt detection with the short-lived radioactive gases.
Sem. Nucl. Med. 10: 27-38, 1980.

205. Watson,D.D., Kenny,P.J., Janowitz,W.R., Tamer,D.M., Gilson,A.J.: Detection of left-to-right shunts by inhalation of Oxygen-15-labeled carbon dioxide.
In: Nuclear Cardiology: Principles and Methods (eds.: A.N.Serafini, A.J.Gilson, W.M.Smoak), Plenum Medical Book Company, New York, London: 49-63, 1977.

206. Wegner, P.: Programming with ADA, an introduction by means of graduated examples.
Prentice-Hall, Inc., Englewood Cliffs, N.J. 07632, 1980.

207. Wessler, S.: Factors in the initiation of deep venous thrombosis. In: Thromboembolism, Ätiology, Advances in prevention and management (ed. Nicolaides, A.N.),
Med. and Techn. Publishing Co., Lancaster: 9-28,1975.

208. Westermann, K., Trentz, O., Pretschner, P., Mellmann, J., Reuter, Th.: Medikamentöse Thromboembolieprophylaxe bei hüftchirurgischen Eingriffen. In: Postop. Thromboembolie-Prophylaxe (Hrsg. Pabst, H.W., Maurer, G.),
F.K. Schattauer-Verlag, Stuttgart, New York: 145-154, 1977.

209. Wexler, J.P., Blaufox, M.D.: Radionuclide evaluation of left ventricular performance with nonimaging probes.
Semin. Nucl. Med. 9: 310-319, 1979.

210. Wickham, K.: PASCAL im Vergleich mit anderen Progammiersprachen. Elektronik 29: 47-54, 1980.

211. Wirth, N.: Algorithms + data structures = programs. Prentice-Hall, Inc., Englewood Cliffs, N.J., 1976.

212. Wirth, N.: A personal computer based on a high-level language. In: Language design and programming methodology (ed. Tobias, J.M.), Bd. 79, Springer-Verlag, Berlin, Heidelberg, New York: 191-193, 1980.

213. Wirth, N.: The module: a system structuring facility in high-level programming languages. In: Language design and programming methodology (ed. Tobias, J.M.), Bd. 79, Springer-Verlag, Berlin, Heidelberg, New York: 1-24, 1980.

214. Wolf, H.: Lineare Systeme und Netzwerke. Springer-Verlag, Berlin, Heidelberg, New York, 1971.

215. Wunsch, G.: Systemanalyse. Bd. 1: Lineare Systeme, 2. Aufl. Dr. A. Hüthig Verlag, Heidelberg, Mainz, Basel, 1971.

216. Wuppermann, Th., Mellmann, J., Jarosch von Schweder, J.: Morphometric characteristics of incompetent perforating veins in primary varicosis of the lower leg. VASA 7: 66-70, 1978.

217. Wuppermann, Th., Mellmann, J., Fröhlich, H.: Experimentelle und phlebographische Befunde zur chronisch-venösen Insuffizienz. Der Hautarzt 30: 186-191, 1979.

218. Zählrohre 1977. Valvo Handbuch, Hamburg, 1977.

219. Zanio, K. Akutagawa, W., Montano, H.: Analysis of CdTe probes. IEEE Trans. Nucl. Sci., NS-19: 257-262, 1972.

220. Zierler, K.L.: Equations for measuring blood flow by external monitoring of radioisotopes. Circ. Res. 16: 309-321, 1965.

8. INDEX

APPENDIX

An engymetric detector system as described in this book is manufactured and sold by the SIEMENS Medical Engineering Group under the name "ENGYPAN".

The SIEMENS ENGYPAN SYSTEM includes the software for the analysis of engymetric time-activity-histograms (DISYA), as described in section 3.3.

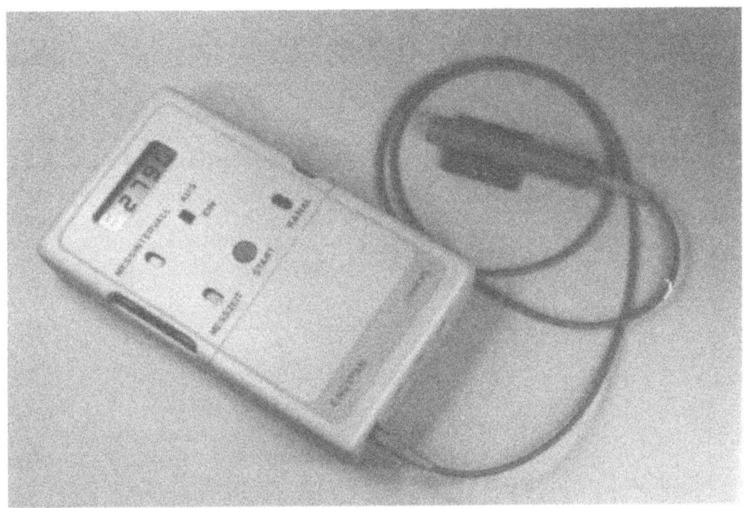

SIEMENS ENGYPAN selectable detector preamplifier and 4-channel storage device combined into a wearable unit. An 8 mm GM-tube is used as the detector in the model illustrated.

Technical Data

Number of detector channels	:	4
Sixteen-step time interval range	:	0.5 s - 286 min
Number of intervals/channel	:	64

Battery powered

CMOS technology

Medizinische Informatik und Statistik

Band 13: S. Biefang, W. Köpcke und M. A. Schreiber, Manual für die Planung und Durchführung von Therapiestudien. IV, 92 Seiten. 1979.

Band 14: Datenpräsentation. Frühjahrstagung, Heidelberg 1979. Herausgegeben von J. R. Möhr und C. O. Köhler. XVI, 318 Seiten. 1979.

Band 15: Probleme einer systematischen Früherkennung. 6. Frühjahrstagung, Heidelberg 1979. Herausgegeben von W. van Eimeren und A. Neiß. VI, 176 Seiten, 1979.

Band 16: Informationsverarbeitung in der Medizin -Wege und Irrwege-. Herausgegeben von C. Th. Ehlers und R. Klar. XI, 796 Seiten. 1980.

Band 17: Biometrie – heute und morgen. Interregionales Biometrisches Kolloquium 1980. Herausgegeben von W. Köpcke und K. Überla. X, 369 Seiten. 1980.

Band 18: R. Fischer, Automatische Schreibfehlerkorrektur in Texten. Anwendung auf ein medizinisches Lexikon. X, 89 Seiten. 1980.

Band 19: H. J. Rath, Peristaltische Strömungen. VIII, 119 Seiten. 1980.

Band 20: Robuste Verfahren. 25. Biometrisches Kolloquium der Deutschen Region der Internationalen Biometrischen Gesellschaft, Bad Nauheim, März 1979. Herausgegeben von H. Nowak und R. Zentgraf. V, 121 Seiten. 1980.

Band 21: Betriebsärztliche Informationssysteme. Frühjahrstagung, München, 1980. Herausgegeben von J. R. Möhr und C. O. Köhler. XI, 183 Seiten. 1980.

Band 22: Modelle in der Medizin. Theorie und Praxis. Herausgegeben von H. J. Jesdinsky und V. Weidtman. XIX, 786 Seiten. 1980.

Band 23: Th. Kriedel, Effizienzanalysen von Gesundheitsprojekten. Diskussion und Andwendung auf Epilepsieambulanzen. XI, 287 Seiten. 1980.

Band 24: G. K. Wolf, Klinische Forschung mittels verteilungsunabhangiger Methoden. X, 141 Seiten. 1980.

Band 25: Ausbildung in Medizinischer Dokumentation, Statistik und Datenverarbeitung. Herausgegeben von W. Gaus. X, 122 Seiten. 19.

Band 26: Explorative Datenanalyse. Frühjahrstagung, München, 1980. Herausgegeben von N. Victor, W. Lehmacher und W. van Eimeren. Wolf 1 Seiten. 1980.

Band 27: Systeme und Signalverarbeitung in der Nuklearmedizin. Proceedings. Herausgegeben von S. J. Pöppl und D. P. Pretschner. IX, 317 Seiten. 1981.

Band 28: Nachsorge und Krankheitsverlaufsanalyse. 25. Jahrestagung der GMDS, Erlangen, September 1980. Herausgegeben von L. Horbach und C. Duhme. XII, 697 Seiten. 1981.

Band 29: Datenquellen für Sozialmedizin und Epidemiologie. Herausgegeben von Ralph Brennecke, Eberhard Greiser, Helmut A. Paul und Elisabeth Schach. VIII, 277 Seiten. 1981.

Band 30: D. Möller, Ein geschlossenes nichtlineares Modell zur Simulation des Kurzzeitverhaltens des Kreislaufsystems und seine Anwendung zur Identifikation. XV, 225 Seiten. 1981.

Band 31: Qualitätssicherung in der Medizin. Probleme und Lösungsansätze. GMDS-Frühjahrstagung, Tübingen, 1981. Herausgegeben von H. K. Selbmann, F. W. Schwartz und W. van Eimeren. VII, 199 Seiten. 1981.

Band 32: Otto Richter, Mathematische Modelle für die klinische Forschung: enzymatische und pharmakokinetische Prozesse. IX, 196 Seiten. 1981.

Band 33: Therapiestudien. 26. Jahrestagung der GMDS, Gießen, September 1981. Herausgegeben von N. Victor, J. Dudeck und E. P. Broszio. VII, 600 Seiten. 1981.

Band 34: C. E. M. Dietrich, P. Walleitner, Warteschlangen-Theorie und Gesundheitswesen. VIII, 96 Seiten 1982.

GPSR Compliance
The European Union's (EU) General Product Safety Regulation (GPSR) is a set of rules that requires consumer products to be safe and our obligations to ensure this.

If you have any concerns about our products, you can contact us on

ProductSafety@springernature.com

In case Publisher is established outside the EU, the EU authorized representative is:

Springer Nature Customer Service Center GmbH
Europaplatz 3
69115 Heidelberg, Germany

www.ingramcontent.com/pod-product-compliance
Ingram Content Group UK Ltd.
Pitfield, Milton Keynes, MK11 3LW, UK
UKHW061656190726
13853UKWH00008B/2245

* 9 7 8 3 6 4 2 9 3 2 2 1 2 *